THE
YUM
FACTOR

Changing Your Attitude
Toward Food and Fitness

LISA NATOLI AND JEANINE BARONE

authorHOUSE®

AuthorHouse™
1663 Liberty Drive
Bloomington, IN 47403
www.authorhouse.com
Phone: 1 (800) 839-8640

Published by AuthorHouse 08/05/2019

ISBN: 978-1-7283-1445-7 (sc)
ISBN: 978-1-7283-1444-0 (e)

Library of Congress Control Number: 2019906513

The Yum Factor Philosophy:
Eating should be enjoyable and fitness should be fun.

TABLE OF CONTENTS

PREFACE

I have struggled with my weight almost my entire life. My name is Lisa Natoli, and I am a minister and spiritual teacher living in Maine. In 2016, I lost 60 pounds – all without dieting, counting calories or measuring food. How did I do it? By changing my thoughts and attitude about not only food and fitness, but more importantly about how I live and how I think. I wrote this book with my friend Jeanine Barone, who is a nutritionist and exercise physiologist. These pages contain all the wisdom and advice that Jeanine gave me over a three-year period of weekly counseling sessions that helped me to transform my body, my mind and my life.

Our goal in this book is to inspire you to make a similar change in your relationship with yourself and with food and fitness. We call our philosophy Food/Fit/Aware, and we've divided the book into these three sections (though you'll notice a lot of the ideas and sections overlap and intersect). By sharing our ideas, we hope to inspire you to love yourself, to be healthy and active, to get out into nature a little more every day and to live a vibrant, joyful life that you love.

INTRODUCTION

Imagine living a life you love, in a body that is fit, healthy and active. Well, guess what? It's totally possible. I'm here to share with you the big secret of finding success when it comes to transforming your life and body, to getting balanced and being connected in a way that makes you feel vibrant, alive and grateful.

The secret is this: There is no secret. There is no grand plan. No one-size-fits-all.

Most people think they need to drop a bunch of weight and THEN they can begin living healthy. They believe the best route is to do something radical just to get started, and then somehow transition to a healthy lifestyle. We say: Skip the radical weight loss part and move over to the healthy living part now. It's time to get yourself unstuck from the idea that your life will start later, once your body magically transforms. This book is designed to inspire and encourage you to live a vibrant, healthy and active life NOW. These chapters contain ideas, practices, steps and actions that you can take now to help you feel that every day is amazing, beautiful and fun, and to lift you up out of the rut of diet mentality.

We know there is a whole lot of contradictory information out there about eating healthy. After debating whether we wanted to say anything about it here in this book, or give an actual food program, we decided against it. What ends up happening is that the second you give someone a food plan or food rules it becomes a religion, or a magical plan to melt off the pounds. And that is not what this book is about.

In the beginning, I kept asking Jeanine for a food plan or a program that I could follow, and she wouldn't give me one. She never did. Yet, three years later I had dropped 60 pounds and was feeling more active and fit than in at least 20 years. That's why there is no plan or program in this book — because we truly believe that everyone instinctively and intuitively knows which foods support great health and which do not.

Think about what kinds of foods you typically eat now. How do you feel while you are eating? How do you feel after you eat? It's our observation that most people are unconscious and on automatic pilot, not aware of how they feel before, during and after eating.

We want you to find your own way, to get to know your own mind, your own needs, your own body. Everyone is different and therefore giving a one-size-fits-all food program just doesn't work. Believe it or not, you are going to be your own guru at figuring out what you need to eat to live your best life!

That's probably not what you want to hear. Many people I've met who have seen my weight loss simply want me to tell them what I eat so they can eat that way too. They want to know what I have for breakfast, lunch, dinner and snacks. When I tell them what I eat, they get a confused look on their faces because there is no formula, no method. Sure, I eat healthy, but then I also have moments when I eat things not considered healthy — so listing what I eat doesn't work because it's not about the food. But then again, it *is* about the food! It's a bit of a paradox. It's about understanding your relationship with yourself and the food you eat. That's how you change.

This is NOT a diet and we are not focusing on weight loss. This is about being healthy, fit, vibrant, active and alive. It's about enjoying food and enjoying life. Eating healthy and caring for your body (and caring for your life!) is all about your attitude and state of mind. Most people are living in guilt all the time because they set up strict rules for themselves which are impossible to attain. Changing your mindset is going to require some radical honesty. If you want to live a vibrant life, you will need to start discovering what makes you feel good and what makes you feel not so good.

In today's fast-paced, digital information society, we are bombarded every day with the latest quick-fix, practical tips and tools to feel better, to be more productive, to accomplish more. I'm not here to announce fancy techniques or a newly discovered hidden secret guaranteed to magically transform your life and body in five easy steps. I am not going to promise you a life that will get better later. The bottom line is that "later" is the problem — *there is no later.* That's the carrot that dangles in front of everyone who has ever dieted, with promises of a brighter tomorrow. As you've probably already discovered through endless dieting, that doesn't work.

The whole difficulty (and trap, if you ask me) with diets, weight-loss techniques and exercise programs is that they promise a different, improved, happier you... later. But here is the thing: You are whole and perfect right now, right in this moment. When you realize this simple truth, you start caring about yourself, you decide to be healthy and active and you naturally start making different food and fitness choices that are in alignment with honoring and embracing yourself.

Most people flat-out reject this idea and deny it by offering "proof" of how this statement does not apply to them. They say there is no such thing as perfect, that no one is perfect. But you *are* perfect in your imperfection. You are good enough just the way you are right now. Soak that in. You are good enough now. You are worthy of a magnificent, beautiful life that is all yours.

Imagine if you were to begin treating yourself with kindness, respect and love instead of constantly berating and condemning yourself. Imagine what a gift it would be to yourself if you decided to stop beating yourself up for excess weight, an inactive lifestyle, missed opportunities and a life that has passed you by. Imagine empowering yourself enough that you could do away with victim mentality and negative thinking. Wouldn't that be awesome?

Even though we live in a world with so much information and knowledge for improving our lives right at our fingertips, most people are worse off than ever before. The conflict in the world and in people's minds is at an all-time high. How can this be? How did we become a society of people so disconnected from each other and, more importantly, disconnected from ourselves, our own bodies, our own lives? With all our electronic devices, we have become a civilization that is externally focused. We've lost our connection with simplicity, with nature, with life itself and with love. This is the big secret to transformation: Love yourself.

Shocking, I know. It can't possibly be that simple, and yet in all my work as a spiritual teacher I have found that this two-word-instruction — "love yourself" — is perhaps the most difficult thing for people to do. And that, of course, is the whole problem. The difficulties you experience in weight loss and elsewhere in life can often be chalked up to the fact that you don't truly know yourself, and you don't truly love yourself.

We all run around trying to find ways to be happy, to improve ourselves, to make money, to be successful, to stay on top of things. And we exert a tremendous amount of energy trying to change our appearance, our health, our bodies, our relationships — anything to feel complete and whole. But somehow, we still keep missing the mark. We take workshops and online classes and buy books that promise us a happy life, and halfway through we realize this isn't it. So, we buy the next online course, or try the latest new workout craze in the hopes that maybe this one is the one. And it never is. Anything that promises success "later" at some point in the future is always destined to fail. Don't waste your money. Don't waste your time.

Why is this? Because you ARE THERE already. This is your life now. This is it. This is what it looks like, in all its splendor. You've been given a beautiful gift in every day that you wake up, and you are missing it completely by focusing on how horrible you are, how terrible your life is, how much weight you've gained. You're missing the whole point of it! Life is meant to be fun, an adventure, a time of wonder and curiosity and connection with yourself and others. It's time to break the cycle, to stop running around with the false belief that your life will start later. Your life is happening now. This is it.

Transformation begins when you open your eyes and see yourself and your life differently in a new way. A life of joy comes from balance, from slowing down, from going outside in nature, from being truly connected within to your fundamental needs, wants and purpose in life. It comes from accepting yourself and loving yourself and being kind to yourself.

I know this all sounds very basic, but look around — almost no one is doing it. In my work as a spiritual teacher, I have met thousands of people who have tons of knowledge and years of devotion but who self-sabotage on a daily (hourly!) basis. I WAS one of those people, and in this book, you will learn my story and how I changed all that.

For me, developing awareness was the key to breaking out of years of self-sabotage — a prison of my own making. Awareness is a great gift — you see things in a new way. I came to an awareness of my relationship with food, awareness of my thought patterns, awareness of my feelings and emotions, awareness of my hidden self-hatred, awareness of my guilt, shame and disappointment. (It's shocking at first when you realize how much you attack yourself with your own thinking.)

And then came the final level of awareness: a realization of how powerful I am to change my own mind and walk away from negative thought processes. Awareness of how, if I didn't start taking care of myself, my whole life was going to pass me by in a body that was overweight and slow-moving. I didn't want to miss another second!

Our goal in this book is to inspire you to change your relationship with yourself and with food and fitness. We call our philosophy Food/Fit/Aware: It's the practice of being aware of what you eat, how you eat, how you move, how you think and how you feel. We'll coach you on how to go within, how to pay close attention to your thought patterns, in order to discover both what's holding you back, and what can move you forward. I know this sounds like a cliché — go within — but seriously, it is crucially important to decide to have moments of quiet and stillness as a regular practice, so you can begin to see all the unconscious patterns and programs that are running the show in your life. You will find that you can begin changing your life today, and that you can immediately begin to feel better. (You might already feel better just from reading this Introduction.) This is our hope — that you see new possibilities for yourself. That you stop dieting. That you stop with the crazy gadgets and packaged programs promising to make you a "better" version of yourself. That you stop torturing yourself with ideas of deprivation, thinking it's the only way to reach your goal. Deprivation never led anyone to a happy life — it might have gotten some people to drop weight, but it's no way to live.

Bottom line: You don't have to suffer anymore. You can have your cake and eat it too.

The biggest turning point in my journey came about two years into my work with Jeanine, when she came to a simple realization: that *I didn't want to change.* I can remember the day like it was this morning. I had been telling her every week how much I wanted to change, that I was committed to change and that I would do anything it took to change. I would make small tweaks in my thinking, eating and exercise, but nothing budged. My weight remained the same. My habits remained the same. As much as I said the words "I want to change," these words only scratched the surface. They hadn't sunk deep down into my heart and mind, into the very core of my being — and so the cycle continued. Until one day, Jeanine said to me: "Lisa, you don't want to change. I'm not working with you anymore. We are not doing this. We're done. This is a waste of my time."

Her words were a jolt and a wake-up call — deep down, I knew she was right. And that's the day change began to occur.

Many people say they want to change, but very few mean it. They are really just hoping that someone will come along with a magic wand or a magic pill or a magic powder — or a magic diet — to make their lives wonderful without having to actually change their way of doing things. So, you need to ask yourself honestly: Do I really want to change? Am I ready to change my way of living, my attitude, my words and most importantly, my way of thinking?

If your answer is "Yes, absolutely, immediately!" it must be more than just words. You must really mean it. You must be ready to overhaul your life. That might sound dramatic, but if you want to see real change, it's going to take a drastic transformation in your attitude, in the way you do things, in the very way you think about yourself and your life. If you want to start living a life of joy, wonder and curiosity, in a body that is fit and healthy, you can't keep going along the way you have been. It's that simple.

So, ask yourself: Do I really want to change? Am I ready to choose and create a different, better life? Am I willing to change my thinking, attitude and habits? If the answer is YES, then let's go!

LISA'S STORY

I have been a professional teacher of healing and transformation since 2000, and yet I somehow could not see my own blind spots when it came to health, food and fitness. I was overeating, overweight, and overtired.

In truth, I could see what I was doing — on some level I was aware of my own self-sabotage, self-hatred and attack thoughts — but I did nothing to change it. I was teaching workshops around the world, helping people to notice their thoughts and feelings — and with my guidance thousands of people were experiencing breakthroughs, healing and change. Helping people gave me great fulfillment, and I thought of myself as a happy person. Yet I overate. I wasn't active. I would feel guilty. Then I would beat myself up about my lack of discipline and promise myself to start eating healthier, to be more conscious. This vicious cycle went on for years.

What I have noticed in my work as a spiritual teacher is that often (practically 10 times out of 10) it takes another person to point out things that we cannot see in ourselves. After we began our weekly counseling sessions, it was Jeanine who pointed out my inner negativity and self-sabotage — and even then, it was a long time before I truly recognized what I was doing to myself. She would say "Wow, Lisa, I can't believe the way you talk about yourself" and I would say "Yes, wow. You're right." And then I wouldn't do anything about it. I'd keep thinking self-hating thoughts, believing that sticking to a diet would change me. This went on for about a year, and all the while Jeanine continued to point out to me my negative self-talk on the phone. But I just couldn't see it. This is how unconscious we are in certain areas of our lives. I had dedicated my life to teaching people how to watch their thoughts, words and emotions, and yet I wasn't doing it myself. I spent my days reminding people of their perfection and wholeness, working hard to inspire others with my radio show, videos and online courses, changing people's lives around the world — all the while continuing to hate myself.

I started gaining weight when I was about 11 or 12 years old and I have been on every possible diet known to man since then. Before then I was an active, healthy, happy little kid with no food issues, who wasn't even conscious of her body. I played outside all the time, wasn't all that interested in meals, wasn't concerned with eating everything on my plate. I just wanted to get back to playing outside or reading a book. I had no self-esteem issues. No body issues.

But all that started changing when I hit 11 or 12. I remember being at summer camp, where some of the older boys started paying attention to me and I didn't like it. I didn't like it at all. Before that I used to stay outside all day long playing, reading, biking, swimming, doing cartwheels on the front lawn, walking in the woods, completely free — until those boys began coming around and flirting with me. I felt nervous and uncomfortable, so I began to stay inside. I began isolating myself and hiding. Shortly after this I started snacking and piling food on my plate and wanting second helpings. Suddenly food became a comfort and friend to me, and I started gaining weight.

It's my belief that we all can find out when the disconnect began in our lives, when we began to become self-conscious and at the same time go unconscious. When did you lose your zest for life? When did you stop playing? When did you start hiding? When did you start becoming afraid? Can you remember? I don't think it's necessary to go on a hunt through your childhood to find out exactly when things went off the grid: It's enough simply to become aware that, if you are unhappy, overweight and unhealthy, then at some point, somewhere, there was a disconnect.

It was Jeanine who helped me to recognize all this, to examine the reasons for my unconscious eating habits and negative self-talk. She also inspired me to see things in a new way, so I could move past these patterns. You will love her.

This book is a result of all her inspiration, guidance and direction. It might sound dramatic to say, but she woke me up from sleepwalking through life.

Jeanine and I have been friends since 1992, when I was hired as an assistant to the Associate Publisher at an NYC publishing office where she worked in editorial as a health writer and researcher. She is one of the smartest, funniest and most fascinating people I know — and one of the most eclectic. Yes, she's a nutritionist and exercise physiologist; but she's also a travel, food and health writer, photographer, comedy screenwriter, and product/fashion designer. She designs travel bags, quirky dolls and clothing for the savvy traveler; she loves taking photographs (most of the gorgeous photos in this book are hers); and her greatest passion is going on travel adventures and finding off-the-beaten track places that most people never visit. She has an extremely curious mind, with an "I wonder" attitude. (I wonder what's around that corner? I wonder if I can find an interesting restaurant? I wonder where that trail leads?) She loves hiking, biking, Nordic skiing, and jump roping. She loves food, but gourmet stuff that's made with love, like handmade dark chocolates with unusual ingredients. She is an explorer in the true sense of the word.

In 2000, I was laid off from my publishing job due to organizational restructuring. This turned out to be the best thing that could have ever happened to me. Even though I loved all my years working there, I hadn't been happy for a while. With no job and no ties to New York anymore, I moved to Wisconsin in a spur-of-the-moment decision to enroll in an Academy that was dedicated to A Course in Miracles. It was originally supposed to be just a 30-day retreat, but as soon as I arrived there I knew I wanted to stay. I went back to New York, packed up my apartment, gave almost everything away and said goodbye to the city. Over the next several years, I saw Jeanine off and on, but it was harder to stay close now that we weren't in the same town. Starting around 2008, we realized our friendship was important and that too much time had passed without seeing each other — so we made a plan to meet once a year for a week-long vacation together. We missed a couple of years, but mostly we kept our promise to each other.

Over 25 years of friendship, Jeanine has patiently watched me go through all my different diet phases — Slimfast, Atkins, Weight Watchers, vegetarian, protein powder shakes, meal replacement shakes, low carb, raw food, vegan, paleo, clean. I've tried it all. Every time I would tell her about my latest diet, her response was always the same: "Oh boy."

Now here's the thing: Jeanine has a hard-core science background in nutrition and exercise. She knows that quick-fixes don't work. Sometimes, in exasperation, she would say "Lisa!" and then give the same speech about what works, based on scientific research and not some fad: Eat healthy, don't eat huge portions, pay attention to how you feel, eat colorfully, be active. "This is not rocket science," she would say. "This is a way of eating, a way of living, a lifestyle change, not a diet, not something you go on and then off." It all sounded good — the slow and steady approach — but what I wanted was a fast track to take the weight off as quickly as possible, so that my happy life could begin!

In September 2014, Jeanine and I went on one of our yearly holidays to a convent on the coast of Maine. During that week together, I watched her like a hawk — the way she ate and the way she moved. Meals were buffet style in a dining room, and Jeanine ate whatever she wanted — she truly had no food rules — but I noticed she paid close attention to what went on her plate and what went in her mouth. Also, I noticed she was active all day long, starting with three minutes of jump roping outside every single day. We went on short hikes in the afternoon — not to exercise, but for fun and exploration. What I noticed most was her adventurous spirit and curiosity for discovery. The difference between us, as I saw it, was that she acts on her wonderment, while I often put things off, saying: "I'll do that later." And, of course, later never comes.

After that week, I felt ready to live in a new way. I was frustrated with my weight, which was around the 200-pound mark, so I asked Jeanine for help. We committed to a weekly, 30-minute phone call, with the idea that she would coach me — telling me how she lives and eats and moves — and I would do what she said. During our calls, I wrote down everything — she gave amazing, simple but brilliant advice. But here's the thing: I didn't do what she said, at least not specifically. I made slight changes that were convenient for me, while continuing to hold onto the same patterns and routines. On the sly, I was still dieting — going on fasts and drinking protein shakes and green beverages with expensive powders bought at the health food store. One year passed and nothing changed for me. My weight stayed the same. Jeanine is one of the smartest people I know on the planet, super intuitive to the point of sometimes being scary, so I'm certain she knew back then (without being in my physical presence) that I was doing my own thing and not following her advice. I wanted to believe in her slow-but-steady approach, but I was still holding out for a magic bullet that would miraculously melt off all my excess weight.

If Jeanine was frustrated with me, she didn't outright express it. But I got the sense that she was somehow aware of my private thoughts and behaviors. She just didn't want to push me because the motivation ultimately was going to have to come from within me.

Our next annual trip was the following summer in June 2015: a week-long, 80-mile walking tour along the Nantes-Brest Canal in Brittany, France. Each day, we would walk approximately 10 miles, and each night we would stay in a B&B in a different charming village. We chose the trip because we wanted a holiday that would include being active every day, but the route was flat and not so strenuous that it felt like hard work. On paper, it sounded like a breeze to me: 10 miles a day, walking leisurely on flat ground. How difficult could it be? I thought I was healthy and in good shape. I still hovered around the 200-pound mark, but I felt I carried my weight evenly and that it would be easy.

The first hour of walking showed me a completely different picture. I was sweating, breathing heavily, unable to keep up with Jeanine, and my feet were overheating (I could feel them burning and sweating through my socks). What should have been a breeze quickly turned into my own personal nightmare in the blaring sun, with a backpack full of clothes that got heavier with every step and miles to go ahead of us.

With my self-sabotaging, guilty mind-set still firmly in place, my head filled with shame thoughts like: "If only I had done what Jeanine suggested over the past year — eat healthy and be a little bit active every day — then I'd have the energy to do this now. Instead of this trip being a nightmare, I'd be having a blast, the best time of my life."

I thought I'd been eating healthy with my protein shakes and attempts at dieting. I thought I had changed a little bit over the year, but really, I hadn't changed at all. I hadn't altered my thinking. I still had attack thoughts of blame and shame. I still called myself stupid. I still called myself lazy. I still thought my life was going to start "later," once I dropped some weight. This is the complete opposite of what Jeanine had been coaching me all year — to be gentle to myself, to be kind to myself, to love myself, to honor my body which is a temple for my spirit.

In France, I was faced with the stark reality of my situation. I was overweight, unhealthy, out of shape, with low energy. I was 47 years old and could not walk 15 minutes at a brisk pace without feeling like I needed to sit down and rest for a minute. I realized my goals were no longer about losing weight to look good. This was no longer about "eat less and exercise more." What I needed was a new way of thinking about myself, about food and about being alive.

So, I returned home and continued my weekly 30-minute phone calls with Jeanine. But guess what? I still didn't change! In France, I had my epiphany moment about how different my life could be, how beautiful, how simple — but I came back to the States and picked up right where I left off! I continued to resist everything she said, despite the fact that I was still taking loads of notes and saying to her, "Yes, Yes, Yes. Brilliant, Great idea! Yes, I'll try that." This is how deep my inner patterns and programs ran. It got to the point where I sincerely felt I'd never break the cycle that was so deeply rooted in me: It felt like a big old oak tree with roots growing for 1,000 years. I felt utterly stuck, like nothing was ever going to change for me. I had many days when I thought: "Well, I'm just a food addict. I can't eat normally, like other people. I can't eat like Jeanine. I can't be active."

The turning point, a moment in time I will never forget (and which I mentioned in the Introduction), was a phone call when Jeanine finally said it was time to give up our weekly calls because they were a waste of time. She said it was obvious I had no intention of changing my thinking and there was no point in continuing. That phone call shook me to my core. It woke me up. I DID want to be healthy. I DID want to be active. I DID want to have a fun life, full of curiosity and wonder and adventure. I wanted to get off the dieting-merry-go-round. I realized I was no longer interested in dramatic results or a quick fix. I wanted to change the way I ate and the way I showed up in life because I didn't want to spend the rest of my life feeling the way I had felt for so long: overweight, tired, low energy, frustrated and overwhelmed.

With that phone call, I decided to stop dieting. No more green powder from the health food store that cost $70 a canister. No more attacking myself with negative thoughts. No more body-shaming. It's so interesting how much of the world goes up in arms when people body-shame each other, but no one really notices how much we body-shame ourselves with our own thoughts. What I discovered (and hopefully you will discover it, too) is that when you start to accept yourself as you are now and shift to a place of love, you are able to make changes that seemed impossible before. I had been trying to change myself — by dieting so I could lose weight — so I could feel accepted and loved. But when I reversed the order and moved into acceptance and loving myself as I am now, I naturally started making changes that reflected this love for myself.

When the weight finally did come off (in 2016), it came off so quickly and so effortlessly that many people who knew me thought I must have done something super drastic. One minute I was 200 pounds and what seemed like overnight I was 140. I went from wearing size 14 pants and dresses to size 6 or 8. What most people do NOT know about is the years and years it took to get to the point when I was ready to shift my thinking. People ask me now, "How did you do it?" and the simple truth is: I changed my way of thinking. As soon as I shifted my focus to loving myself, accepting myself and valuing myself, the weight dropped off with little effort at all.

Sure, I made different food choices — largely inspired by the trip to Brittany, which opened my eyes to a new way of living: eating whole fresh food and being an active person. For most of my adult life, my way of eating had involved extremes, all or nothing. I was either dieting (restricted calories, cleanses, depriving myself) or not dieting (eating huge portions of anything and everything). Those were my two speeds and there was no balance, no in-between. By watching how people eat in France — whole fresh foods from nature — and by observing Jeanine, I learned there is a happy medium.

In this book, we'll encourage you to start looking at the reasons YOU want to change, to become more conscious of your inner patterns and motivations. When you are faced with life (and food choices), you'll develop a new habit of asking WHY. Why do you want to change? Are you coming from a place of love (you want to feel better, to be nice to yourself, to be more active and energetic and do fun things)? Or from a place of fear and judgment (you don't like yourself, you're overweight, you want to be loved)?

Another why you'll start asking yourself: Why do you want to eat what you are about to eat? Are you conscious of what is about to go in your mouth? Are you aware of what is on your plate? Are you awake to your food choices? Are you PRESENT for it? You'll develop a practice of pausing before acting/eating. This pause creates a space of silence and stillness which makes all the difference. This, to me, has been one of the greatest lessons I have learned: how to be still before acting. I've learned that I don't have to eat right away. I don't have to react right away, or even react at all anymore. From a place of quiet awareness, I can choose to respond or to do nothing. I don't have to do things NOW, which was a big part of the destructive pattern that led me to overeat — the feeling that I must take care of everything, I must react to everything, I have to stay on top of everything. To know that I can simply RELAX and TRUST and LET GO has been a big part of my healing. I have learned to listen to what I need and what I want. I'm able to feel when I'm full. This is a miracle. I used to eat and eat and eat, and have no connection between my mind and body.

I would shovel food in without any awareness that it might not taste good or that I was already stuffed or that I wasn't even hungry to begin with.

When people ask me how I lost weight and got in shape, this is the short answer: I'm active and I make it a habit to eat really well — food that is whole, fresh and local, rather than processed and from a factory. But the deeper truth is this: Once I started paying attention to and loving myself, I became more receptive to what I needed and wanted. I set out to be healthy and active, and my whole way of living and thinking transformed. The more I came to the quiet space, the more I began to hear my own inner voice guiding me, stopping me when I was full, getting me outside to play and enjoy, leading to me a life of balance.

FOOD

DITCHING THE D-WORD

I really love food. I love cooking food, shopping for food, talking about food. I love movies about food, chefs, bakeries and restaurants. And most of all: I love eating food. Ask any of my friends and they will tell you that I'm the one who wants to talk about what I ate for breakfast, what I plan to eat for lunch and dinner and what we can eat tomorrow. I love cookbooks. I love being in the kitchen. I love going out to eat. I love bringing a casserole or a dessert to a party. Sometimes when I'm eating a meal by myself, I'll Google recipes to see how other people make the same dish. For example, while eating baked macaroni and cheese made from my mom's recipe, I'll sit in front of the computer searching for mac and cheese recipes from five-star chefs. Then later that week, I'll test out one of their recipes.

I'm also fascinated by the social element of food — how it brings people together. When I was 16, still in high school, I started throwing parties for my friends. I loved gathering people around a table. In 1988, I got my first degree in Burlington, Vermont — an Associates of Science degree in hotel/restaurant management. My dream was to someday open up a B&B where I would serve people delicious meals and make them happy. It was my vision to give people an unforgettable experience and in my vision, food was always involved.

Over the years, long after I moved on from that initial dream, my fascination with food persisted. I'm always curious about what my friends, family or even strangers at a restaurant are eating. I find it to be a great conversation starter. When we were visiting my husband's five-year-old granddaughter, Lily, in Texas, she said, "Lisa, you know what's WEIRD??? You always want to know what I ate! It's so weird!" Five years old, and she was on to me. It's true. My love for food is that transparent. I want details. I want descriptions. Totally crazy, right? Well, turns out a lot of people are like me and do the same thing.

This is why the approach in this book works so wonderfully for me, and why dieting was always a disaster: because I love food. I am fascinated by it. I'm thrilled by it — that you can start with a seed and grow it into something with thousands of different variations of tastes and textures — something that you can eat, that will nourish you. So going on a diet, with all its restrictions, always felt like a jail sentence to me. There was no fun in that. No pleasure. No joy. With the Food/Fit/Aware approach, nothing is off-limits, ever. I never deprive myself or restrict myself — I make food choices all over the map. What Jeanine taught me is how to find a style of eating that I can live with for the long term. She taught me how to see myself differently, so that I don't even want to eat second helpings and huge portions anymore.

Because of this love of food, and my inner drive that equates food with love, a lot of issues came up for me every time I went on a diet and tried to get in shape. I would try to stop thinking about meals, to shut off my love for food and curiosity about it. I would stop cooking, and go on some program that almost always involved cutting myself off from my social circle and limiting my food intake. A diet, by definition, involves deprivation — it's something you're meant to go on, lose weight and then go off again. And every time, I would find myself having to explain my diet to friends and family, over and over again:

Why can't you come out to eat with us? I'm on a diet.

Why are you just ordering a salad? I'm on a diet.

Why aren't you ordering dessert? I'm on a diet.

But the truth is, food *should* taste good and you don
yourself. So, ditch the D-word: You can stop dicting. You
And you can still get fit and healthy. That's why this
Yum Factor!

What you put in your mouth should be delicious and Yum. Try this fun
exercise: Every time you eat something, ask yourself if it makes you say or
think "Yum!" If it's not totally Yum and delicious, then ask yourself "Why
am I eating this?"

By the same token, if you aren't hungry but you're still eating, ask yourself
"Why am I eating this?" Often, we eat food just because it's around, or
because we're bored or stressed out. We have lots of reasons that have
nothing to do with hunger. Maybe we've even lost touch with what being
hungry really feels like.

And what makes it worse, many of us choose foods that are packaged,
processed and cheap because we think we can't afford to eat healthy. We
load up on food that has very little nutritional value and then wonder why
we're still hungry and not satisfied. (What's curious about this one is that
many people don't think twice about spending money on packaged diet
foods, powders and programs.)

Why are you eating what you eat? Instead of going on a diet, simply start
to pay closer attention to yourself, to your thinking, to your habits, to
your behavior that may have become unconscious — it's a great place to
start. Begin to notice how you feel when you eat. Do you even LIKE what
you're eating? Does it taste good? Are you happy? Are you present in the
moment? Are you enjoying your eating experience?

While traveling with Jeanine in Brittany on our one-week hiking trip in
2015, I noticed that almost everything we ate was fresh, locally sourced and
delicious. There were no particular food rules, but there was also very little
in the way of processed items. We ate fresh bread, cheese, meat, butter (all
in moderate quantities), as well as fruits and vegetables. We sat down for
every meal, and it felt like a mini-holiday three times a day.

y morning we had homemade yogurt with berries straight from omeone's garden, freshly picked that morning or the day before. Yum! Yum! Yum! The Yum Factor was off the charts. We ate croissants that came straight from the oven with jam made from fresh strawberries and blueberries picked out of the garden. Portion sizes in France are smaller; by American standards, they might be considered tiny. When a cake was served, most people ate only a bite or two, enjoying it fully. From my observations during our travels, the French don't eat smaller portions because they are dieting; they eat smaller portions because they intuitively understand that you don't need to overeat to feel satisfied.

In France, it's all about quality, not quantity. Eating is about taste and pleasure and leisure. You don't see people snacking mindlessly and you don't see people eating while walking down the street or driving. They don't drink coffee on the go, except maybe a shot of espresso at the bar en route to work. (And they drink it while standing at the counter, fully present for the experience.) When people in France have a meal, they eat and nothing else. They don't text. They don't scroll on the computer. They eat. It's them and the food with no distractions. Sometimes, dinner can be one to two hours long.

After I had dropped 60 pounds in what seemed like a completely effortless way, I asked my husband Bill what he thought changed for me this time around. I thought he would be a great person to ask, since he has watched me through countless new food plans for the past six years. He thought carefully about his answer, and then he said: "You stopped dieting. You started eating healthy and smaller portions." I loved his answer because I had not discussed any of the contents of this book with him. He didn't know that no foods were off limits. But, it was obvious to him that my focus and attitude had changed.

One of the very first things Jeanine told me when we began having our weekly counseling calls was to banish the word "diet" from my vocabulary. This instruction included the use of any "food program" phrases that were restrictive to a particular kind of food — phrases like raw, vegan, low-carb, plant-based, vegetarian, clean, gluten-free, no-sugar and no-flour.

Despite this advice, for the first year I couldn't stop dieting. I still felt like I needed a plan or program to follow, that there was no way to manage my eating without some kind of external guidelines. My experience for most of my life was that a bowl of ice cream or a slice of pizza would trigger me to go completely out of control. I felt powerless around chocolate — which is crazy to me now — and a piece of chocolate could cause me to blank out and go overboard for a week. But this was my experience, and so I felt I needed to be in absolute control at all times. Since this is literally impossible, it was all or nothing, cycling back and forth, again and again.

Jeanine knew from the very beginning that my weight wasn't the real issue. I wanted to lose 40 pounds, but she told me to forget about losing weight and to focus instead on being conscious, making small deliberate choices about what I put in my mouth, and moving my body a little bit more, just slight changes every day. She said, "Once you change your mind and attitude, you will choose foods appropriately and it won't be a diet."

It took me a long time to trust Jeanine and her advice, which really meant that it took me a long time to trust myself. When I finally did, I began to let go of the food programs. I decided to feel good and to eat foods that made me feel good. This meant being able to eat whatever I want, but also paying attention to how I felt during and after eating. Does eating a gigantic piece of cake make me feel good? Not really. Slowly but steadily, I began to make different food choices.

Since I lost the weight, "What do you eat?" is the #1 question I get asked. Here is my answer: I eat whatever I want. That is the truth. Quite often, the response is "No, really. What do you eat EXACTLY?" People want me to give them a diet, a formula, a plan, but I don't have one. I eat well. I eat healthy. I take care of myself. But then sometimes I indulge and have popcorn at the movies or pizza with friends, and that's taking care of myself too. What I don't do anymore is eat a whole pizza mindlessly at home. I pay attention to what my mind is doing before I put anything in my mouth. I'm conscious to what I am doing, what I am thinking, what I am about to eat, and why.

I love meals that are delicious and healthy. If I look at a food label and it has sugar as the first or second ingredient or if it has ingredients that are unrecognizable, I don't eat it. Why would you eat something if you have no clue what it is? Instead, I prefer to eat food that is food. I love food that is fresh, preferably grown from the earth, not from a package or a can or processed in a factory. I love foods that are packed with nutrients, rather than additives. I eat meat, fish, eggs and chicken and I do my best to buy local. I aim for fresh and homemade, with a high Yum Factor.

Diets are about deprivation, obsession and manipulation: counting calories, measuring, calculating (next meal, fat grams, protein).

Diets are about guilt. Foods are labeled "good" or "bad," and some are off limits entirely. You feel terrible about eating, punishing yourself now in order to achieve some goal in the future. That's no way to live.

Diets are something you go on and go off, not a way of living.

And let's be real here: Diets are a form of torture. I think we can all agree on this point.

You can stop dieting. Food is not the enemy. Food is delicious and fun. Food is your friend.

A WORD FROM JEANINE

When you go on a diet, almost by definition, it means you'll be going off that diet one day. Sure, on the short term, you'll likely lose weight, no matter what diet you follow. But studies have found that more than 90% of dieters fail, regaining the weight they lost, and then some. Diets don't work over the long term because a combination of genetic, metabolic, hormonal, neurological and psychological factors all come into play, almost conspiring to maintain your body weight. One common effect that may occur in dieters is that they spend more time thinking about and seeking food, feeling an enormous reward when they eat, but then not really being satisfied, leading to more food cravings. Another obstacle: Following all the food rules of a diet makes the "don't" foods all that more appealing and difficult to resist.

EATING FOR LIFE

Since my teenage years, carbs and chocolate were my two best friends, my mighty companions. Pasta, bread, candy bars and cake comforted me, soothed me, cheered me up and were generally always there for me. I could depend on them to keep me company, help me over a break-up or give me a sense of celebration whenever I needed a little party or pick-me-up in my day.

But here was the problem: While it's true that carbs and chocolate made me feel good for a little while, afterwards I felt tired. And a little bit (or a lot) guilty. And always wanting more. Some of my favorites were a big bowl of mac and cheese, a few cookies (or the whole bag) or several pieces of toast slathered with butter, sugar and cinnamon (my favorite afternoon snack during high school and college). I would feel happy while eating them (and it wasn't eating so much as scarfing down) but then I would feel tired and lethargic. Usually afterward, I didn't feel like doing much of anything except taking a nap or watching television. These foods did not energize me. Yes, they tasted good, of course. They tasted amazing. I felt joy and giddiness eating pasta swimming in butter with parmesan cheese, a hot bagel with butter and cream cheese, a bowl of ice cream, or a chewy, fudgy brownie. But these foods also generally left me feeling stuffed, unsatisfied and wanting more.

When I decided to ditch dieting, it was because I had started to think in a new way: that my body is perfect just the way it is. I started treating my body like a new car or a temple that needed and deserved my care. It didn't matter that I was almost 200 pounds. I decided to drop the constant criticism — I was going to love myself no matter what. I was done with judging. Done with guilt.

I had made these kinds of declarations in the past, but after a few days I'd find myself falling back into my old unconscious eating patterns, going overboard with donuts, cake, pasta, cheese and everything in sight. Like flipping a switch, I would do a complete reversal: decide that I would "love myself the way I am" and then use this as an excuse to go on a free-for-all.

This time around, it wasn't like that. Instead, with my new state of mind, my focus was on paying attention to and caring for myself. I had a simple, new goal — to live a vibrant life — and to get there I realized I had to find a whole new way of eating. It would have to include two basic ingredients that were important to me: fuel and taste. I was looking for nutrient-dense food that tasted delicious. And after all my years of counseling with Jeanine, I knew where to start: go back to nature. I decided to eat foods as close as possible to their whole and natural state — but they also had to be yummy.

In the early days of living with this new attitude about food, I had no idea how to make it work. "Natural" foods, in my experience, were boring. I could not think of anything duller than a salad with romaine lettuce, tomatoes and chopped up carrots. This was my idea of "healthy," and it was totally unappetizing and unappealing to me.

So, it was time to rethink and relearn everything I thought I knew about nutrition. Over the years, I'd come to believe that "eating healthy" was basically about calories and moderation. Now I started looking at food in terms of nutrients or energy.

My new goal was to live a vibrant life: I no longer cared about losing weight or fitting into a smaller size of jeans. I wanted optimal health. I wanted to feel energized after meals, instead of tired and drained, as had been my experience for much of my life.

I also felt that I needed to find my own way as far as food was concerned, and not just follow another packaged food plan. I didn't care about foods being organic or non-GMO, even though it's what everyone's talking about these days. Everywhere you turn, you hear terms like raw, vegan, Paleo, gluten-free, clean and organic. I don't care about any of that. To me, these are just more labels. It's all just sophisticated diet mumbo-jumbo (and we are ditching diets forever here, right?).

I decided that I was no longer going to let food marketers or diet plans dictate my choices about what is good or bad — no food would be off limits. I needed to figure out what I enjoyed, what tastes I loved, what foods felt good to me and gave my body energy. It was about taste and function.

This wasn't a license to eat anything I wanted, whenever I wanted. It meant that I was going to begin paying attention when I ate, tapping into my senses to find out what was truly enjoyable, while at the same time exploring healthy choices that would fuel my body.

Initially, it was a challenge for me because I thought a plant-based, whole food diet — with fruits, vegetables, seeds and nuts as the main focus — was going to be more like a prison sentence. But, I was determined to figure it out. I kept my goal of "vibrant health" clear in my mind and worked on finding new ways to make my favorite foods more nutritious, with a high Yum Factor. I chose to keep eating fish, chicken and meat, but without adding anything that had been processed or came out of a factory. So, no BBQ Sauce, no gravy out of a package, no pre-made salad dressings.

I cleaned out my refrigerator and cupboards and threw or gave away everything that was canned, boxed or bagged. Anything that had been altered from its original state or with a label on it went into the trash or got donated.

Mostly now, I eat foods in their whole, unprocessed state, as close to nature as possible. Even though I don't "eat organic," I try to avoid chemicals or pesticides and look for organic produce when possible. And here is the key: It has to be totally delicious. The Yum Factor has to be off the charts. Otherwise, what is the point? Meals — and life — are about enjoyment!

I went through a process of trial and error — I knew that I really needed to test out my new way of eating in real life to see first-hand if it made a difference. I decided to give it a full month to see if these changes would produce the benefits I hoped for, if any.

I wish I could say I experienced abundant energy in the first couple of days like some of the "success stories" you read about in all those diet books. But it wasn't like that. I wasn't bouncing out of bed with enthusiasm, but I wasn't dragging out of bed either. I also didn't experience any of the "detoxification" symptoms some people talk about when they shift over to eating natural foods. There was no dramatic transformation, but I still knew that I was never going back to processed factory food. I felt good about fueling my body, which was a whole new and exciting concept for me. So, I stuck with it.

Then I noticed the first big difference: Diminished food cravings. I wasn't hungry all day long anymore. My stomach no longer growled, as it had done for so many years. I didn't have any more of those wild, mood-swing cravings — my energy level felt stable, consistent, even. I wasn't getting tired in the middle of the day. I didn't hear my name being called constantly by the fridge and the cupboards. (I swear, cookies can talk!) Now, in their place, I had only silence in my mind — a feeling of well-being, joy and peace.

Another big benefit developed: I no longer felt the need for gigantic double and triple portions. It was as if my body had stabilized and balanced itself. Eating in this new way, I would start to feel "full" halfway through a meal, and so I would stop eating. That was a major miracle for me!

My love for cooking and being in the kitchen returned and grew: I was determined to only eat food that was totally delicious. I still wanted munchy, crunchy, chocolatey, chewy — so I figured out new and inventive ways to achieve it. Today I make raw cheesecakes from natural ingredients that far surpass any store-bought cake. (I have first-hand evidence for this:

Whenever I bring one of my cakes to a party, it's gone in minutes, while the packaged, store-bought ones sit there practically untouched.)

I also began making homemade soups and desserts with nuts, medjool dates, coconut and cacao. Every afternoon, I made "ice cream" with a frozen banana, cacao powder and unsweetened almond milk. I figured out how to make pasta from zucchini, squash and carrots with a pecan basil garlic sauce with olives that was far more delicious than any mac and cheese I had ever tasted. Sometimes for dinner, my husband Bill would throw a piece of salmon or chicken on the grill and I would make all the sides: quinoa with a raw cashew sauce, chopped up raw spinach or kale, caramelized onions, sweet potatoes cooked in olive oil.

Still, sometimes what I'd really want is a cheeseburger with fries, so I'd have it, and I'd enjoy it. And yes, I still occasionally will eat a piece of cake made with white flour and sugar, or some warm, homemade bread slathered with butter, or my mom's mac and cheese. I'm aware that these foods have no nutritional value whatsoever, but hey, that's okay. And then afterwards, when I feel tired and lethargic, I remember again why I don't eat like this all the time anymore, and get back on track. I still love going out to restaurants, but Bill and I almost always split one meal now. The more in tune I became with myself, the more I realized I didn't need giant portions of food to be satisfied.

When the pounds began falling off me, I didn't notice at first because I wasn't even trying to lose weight. For most of my lifetime of dieting, I was always focused on the numbers on the scale. I used to weigh myself every single day. When my focus changed to my health and happiness, I stopped weighing myself altogether. I put the scale in the cupboard, and didn't think twice. But when a few months later I noticed my clothes hanging looser, I pulled it out again out of curiosity — and saw a 20-pound weight loss.

Being healthy and caring for your life and your body is a mind-set. By obsessing over every little dietary rule and failure — how I lived for most of my life — I was living in daily judgment and guilt. This is no way to live. So instead, concentrate on what your body does for you and how you can support it and fuel it, instead of what it looks like.

I love this new way of eating, this new way of living. I love how my body feels when I fuel it well: strong, healthy and vibrant. I love finding delicious food options that reflect a decision to care for and love myself. I love making food choices that leave me feeling energized and balanced. And you will love it too!

A WORD FROM JEANINE

Eating should be an enjoyable experience, not a labor of counting or measuring. Looking around the world, scientists have identified certain populations who live longer than most — with many healthy people living to be 100 years old — in places such as in Okinawa, Japan, the mountainous interior of Sardinia, Italy, as well as communities of Seventh Day Adventists in Loma Linda, California. (These areas are referred to as the Blue Zones.) Among the factors they all have in common is eating reasonable portions of real food that's as close to the earth as possible, rather than packaged or loaded with added preservatives or sweeteners. Try following the example of these Blue Zone populations — skip the calorie counting and focus on finding fresh foods that you enjoy. Take a look at your plate: If it's colorful — green, red, orange, blue and purple — this generally reflects that it's rich in fresh fruits and vegetables, rather than piled with processed foods that tend to be mostly white, beige and brown. Legumes, nuts and seeds as well as whole grains are also part of balanced eating. If you eat meat, such as beef, pork and lamb, choose lean cuts and make it a side dish, not a main course. Fish (that's not fried) is also a good choice.

FOOD

BEING PRESENT

A lot of books and teachers talk about mindfulness these days. It's everyone's favorite new buzzword, and with good reason. "Mindfulness" is just a fancy way of describing the act of being aware, being conscious, being present while you are doing something. How mindful are you when you are eating? How present? Being "present" is about being in touch with your thoughts when you eat, living in the moment, enjoying food, and paying very close attention to how eating makes you feel.

Before I started working with Jeanine, I would eat unconsciously, without thinking about what I was doing. Becoming present was the key that unlocked the door to ending my lifelong difficulties with food. It seems so simple: Be in touch with your feelings when you eat. But for the longest time I ate like a deprived person, like every meal might be my last. I ate while doing other things — checking email, sending text messages and browsing the internet. I ate to reward myself. And I ate in secret, mostly while driving my car.

I felt hungry almost all of the time. I would wake up hungry. For breakfast, I would eat cereal, toast with eggs, or oatmeal with brown sugar or maple syrup, and an hour later, I would feel like I needed to eat again. For lunch, I would have a sandwich, and an hour later I would be hungry. It was like this all day, so I snacked constantly. Then in the evening, I would eat a huge dinner — meat, vegetables and starches like pasta (I LOVE pasta) with lots of cheese. Still, I would feel hungry afterward, even after a big meal. I went straight from being stuffed to feeling hungry — hunger, as in "I have to eat RIGHT NOW."

When I was a kid, my mom used to panic a little every time I said, "I'm hungry," and felt like she had to feed me on the spot. That attitude passed down to me: At the first sign of hunger, I would think "I need to eat!" and then grab whatever I could and put it in my mouth. Most often it was something quick, sugary and packaged.

Most of the time, I would spend breakfast and lunch in front of the computer — I would never take a proper break for mealtimes. I thought I didn't have time, so I would multi-task: eat at the computer, or while reading a book, or while writing a list of things I had to get done. I was so caught up in my thoughts and to-do list that I didn't pay attention to what went into my mouth. In the evening, dinner was always something heavy — "comfort food" — a reward for my hard work all day long (and still I sometimes worked through dinner).

Cake was another favorite way of rewarding myself. I would spend my days giving energy to other people, but never give anything back to myself in terms of rest and relaxation. So, a couple times a day I would "reward" myself with cake, pasta, toast with butter and jelly or sugar, cookies, chocolate bars, or grilled cheese sandwiches. I saw them all as some kind of a congratulations for a job well done. This was my idea of "taking a break." I never truly congratulated myself for working hard, for the way I was showing up in the world, and so I never truly felt valued.

Another thing I did was to treat food like a "friend" who comforted and soothed me. Sometimes, I would drive to the bakery to "meet" a piece of cake with a coffee. Whenever I felt especially overwhelmed, I HAD to have mac and cheese. In fact, whenever I even SAW mac and cheese, I had to have it. Even if I wasn't hungry, it didn't matter. It was a dish I would eat as a kid and eating it was like visiting with my mom and sisters.

With all these unconscious patterns going on, I noticed almost nothing when I ate. I wasn't PRESENT, tasting and enjoying. A lot of the food

I ate was pretty bland, just covered in butter or cheese. (It's funny to me now how tasteless some of my food choices were.) That's probably why my portions sizes were so gigantic — most of the bites I took weren't truly satisfying as far as taste goes. I didn't notice smells, and I didn't savor my food. I just stuffed it in my mouth, often thinking of second helpings before I even began the first one.

As Jeanine explained to me during our counseling sessions, when we eat for pleasure and enjoyment, all we may really want is the first bite or two and after that, the mind goes unconscious, eating out of habit. Every bite after the first one or two may not be as pleasurable. Most of us don't even notice the first bite, second bite, third bite, fourth bite. We eat a whole plate of food, never realizing we didn't even taste it at all because we weren't really there, we were sleepwalking through the whole thing. So, I decided to wake up and smell the coffee!

I set out to practice being present while I was eating — to pay attention, to notice what I was feeling — and that was my starting point. I began by asking myself during every meal: Am I tasting my food? Am I smelling it? Is it satisfying? What do I love about it? At first, it was like trying to find my way in the dark, but I kept with it. And I repeated to myself: I want to feel good. I want to eat in a way that makes me feel great.

The process was an eye-opener. I woke up to the fact that I was eating almost constantly around the clock, except for when I was sleeping — snacking all day between big meals. I ate when I was hungry, I ate when I wasn't hungry (as a reward or a break). I came to the realization that a lot of what I ate, I didn't even taste because I was paying attention to something else. Now, if I notice my mind distracted and not paying attention to whatever I am eating or drinking, I bring my focus back to the food. I'm present.

I also recognized the fact that, for a long time, eating was the only way I knew how to relax and reward myself. My desire for food gave me a destination — to the grocery store, to the bakery, to a coffee shop — when really, I just wanted a break, period. Now I make sure to take time off for relaxation and enjoyment, without it involving food. Food is no longer my friend or my reward. It's fuel.

Before I began this process, I just accepted the fact that I was hungry all day. The quality of the food I ate didn't matter to me, just the quantity: I thought I needed a LOT of food to get rid of my hunger, so my thinking was "the more, the better." The truth is, I really wasn't hungry, or I didn't need to be – I was just choosing foods that weren't satisfying or energizing. Now, I know what it feels like to really be hungry — when I really need a meal — and I know what it feels like when I'm satisfied. I'm more aware of what's going on in my stomach. I don't keep eating after I'm full.

In fact, the act of being present while I ate had an added benefit as I experimented with new foods and ways of eating: I found my taste buds changed, and heightened. Now, everything matters: taste, freshness, flavor, color, smell. I notice colors a lot now. I gravitate towards foods that look super colorful and vibrant. I go for freshness, for items that look like they were just picked. I'll eat salmon completely plain, but perfectly cooked so that it's flaky with a little bit of a crust on it — no extra sauces, cheese or butter needed, and the Yum Factor is off the charts. I also eat vegetables plain — asparagus, broccoli, baby spinach, red peppers, carrots. I savor the natural taste of these things, with nothing on them.

With this new way of eating, I no longer have dramatic spikes of hunger in that "I'm starving" kind of way. Nothing feels like a food emergency anymore. I usually eat three meals a day, with no snacks, though occasionally between lunch and dinner I might have a raw cookie. Sometimes I'll make a raw dessert for after dinner. When I feel like it, I still do occasionally indulge in treats made with sugar or flour, but afterward I get hungry again almost immediately, just like in the past. So, I just enjoy my few bites, but stay present to the way sugar and flour make my body feel, and know that it's only a treat.

So, at your next meal, concentrate on being mindful and present. When you sit down to eat (if you are even sitting down), how much are you paying attention to what goes in your mouth? Are you mindful of taste, color, texture? Are you present with the food? Are you present with your eating companion? Are your thoughts centered in the present moment?

Think about how much you even like what you are eating. Jeanine has a philosophy that you should LOVE what you are eating — it's got to have a Yum Factor. If the food isn't making you say "Yum!" then why are you eating it? Why do we mindlessly eat things we don't even like? What's up with that? Life is meant to be enjoyed.

When you are about to eat a second helping of food, take the time to ask yourself: Am I really hungry? Or am I bored, stressed, tired or not even thinking about it? Look inside, and become present and aware of how you feel. This one step is so simple, yet so life-changing.

Notice what foods trigger you to want more, more, more — and avoid them. This is what happened to me. I stopped dieting altogether, but I also became aware that some foods trigger me to start eating unconsciously. For me, I learned that it's bread, pasta, white rice, cereal, sugar. So then, with this new awareness (although, let's face it, I had always known these were trigger foods), I started making new decisions.

Now when I eat, I eat. I pay attention to the food, to the experience, to relaxation and enjoyment, to the texture of the food, the color, the aroma. Everything. Even when I drink a coffee, I focus only on drinking the coffee.

As I write this, I'm in Starbucks. A few minutes ago, I had just ordered my usual "tall double cappuccino with almond milk," and then sat down, took off my jacket, opened my computer and was settling in. After they called my name, I walked up to the counter to pick up my coffee, and there it was: a tray of little, individually cut-up brownies in pastel-colored cupcake papers. My mind raced right back to unconscious thinking at that moment. Oh my God! Chocolate cupcakes! And they're free! Yippee!

With my coffee in one hand and a brownie bite in the other, I sat back down. Oh boy! Yay! For a moment, it felt like my birthday, with the unexpected surprise of a cake. But then I touched the brownie. It didn't feel moist and fresh. It felt a little stale, like it might have been sitting out on the counter for a while. "Oh well, it's chocolate, it's free, I have permission! And maybe it's good inside!" I thought.

So, despite all my wisdom and work, I went unconscious. On the one hand, my mind registered that the brownie might be stale, but another part of my brain was already in party-mode. I had almost put it in my mouth before I became present again. "What am I doing?" I knew before even tasting it that I wasn't going to like it. I could tell just from touching and looking at it that it wasn't going to be the absolute best brownie on the planet. So why eat it? What was the point? I put it back in the cupcake wrapper untouched, and it's been sitting here on the table for the last 20 minutes. I'll throw it away later.

I tell you this story to illustrate the fact that even when you've taught yourself to eat mindfully, it still takes work to be present. This morning at Starbucks, I noticed that I didn't really want to eat something, but I almost did it anyway. I just blanked out for a moment. I wasn't here. I wasn't in my body. I wasn't present. And when you are not present, everything happens in a blur — like it's in fast motion — "Brownie! Chocolate! Free! Yay! It's a party!" That's not being present. That's falling back into old unconscious patterns.

Yes, after being on this path for three years, and dropping 60 pounds last year, I still sometimes go unconscious and blank out around food. But once you've practiced and become better at being present while you eat, you will find yourself increasingly able to recognize these moments, and manage them. And the beauty of it is, with every new meal comes another chance to be present — so you can put any slip ups or blank outs into the past.

A WORD FROM JEANINE

Do you ever mindlessly chew and swallow your food, hardly paying attention to its flavor? Do you eat even when you're not hungry, or keep eating until you're uncomfortably full? During meals, are you usually also doing some other activity, like checking email, talking on the phone, or watching TV? The term "mindfulness" has become a buzzword, but it's basically just a term that means being present in the moment. In terms of eating, it means being aware of what's going on internally and externally, both before you eat and during meals. Practicing mindfulness allows you to become aware of your body — what it really feels like to be hungry, satisfied, or full — and also the factors that trigger you to eat. Many studies have found that developing this awareness can help with weight loss. When you eat, that should be your sole activity. Savor your food and be grateful for it. And eat slowly: There's research showing that by slowing down, you'll be more likely to realize when you are full, perhaps because it gives your body time to register and recognize that you are satisfied.

MAKING CHOICES

When you decide to start living as a healthy, happy, active, vibrant person, you need to make choices that reflect that decision. Once you've begun looking inward and becoming aware of your eating habits, you'll figure out what works and what doesn't work for you. With this knowledge, you can begin to make better choices toward your goal of enjoying and appreciating every meal.

In 2017, my husband and I were about to embark on a six-week trip away from home and I had cleaned out the fridge and cupboards. There was literally no food in the house. (This was a rare situation, to not have any food around.) It was the last of the packing and I hadn't eaten in several hours and was hungry. There was a gas station/convenience store as well as a Dunkin Donuts about five miles away, and in the past I would have headed there and bought a bag of nuts or a candy bar or chips or a donut or a bagel with cream cheese. I would have eaten anything, just to get rid of the hunger. But this time I thought, "I don't live that way anymore."

The closest place I could think of to get a great meal was 20 miles away. I knew they made homemade soups and fresh salads there. So, there we went — I would have driven 40 miles if that's what it took. I just don't eat anything anymore unless it's going to be the absolute best and freshest and most delicious. The Yum Factor has to be high, or I won't touch it.

I made that choice to go for the healthier option because I honor myself. I care about myself and I care what I eat. I don't eat junk. Through trial and error, I know that a bagel with cream cheese is only going to make me hungrier than when I started. The store-bought ones don't even taste good. So why eat it? Why bother? I'd rather just have a nice cup of tea or water until I can eat something that is amazing, that will be fuel for my body. I want my body to run optimally and I know what works best for it. I know what foods give me energy and vitality. Once you know how food affects you, you no longer want to sabotage yourself. It's very simple. It's a matter of making decisions, honoring yourself, doing what feels great.

I have discovered that I don't really NEED to eat continuously throughout the day. Being hungry is not a life-or-death situation like I used to believe — I can wait to eat. I no longer want to fill myself with empty calories just because it's the closest and "most convenient." I'll drive an hour to buy the best homemade soups. I've learned to prioritize my time so that I do all the grocery shopping only once a week to stock my kitchen with great food. When I travel, I bring my own food on the plane because I know there's not much that I want to eat in airports. In situations where there is absolutely nothing but packaged food in plastic, I still make it work. If I can't find food that is whole and fresh, I'll have a small portion of something that's not the best choice, but it's all there is at the moment. I get creative. Somehow, I always find something delicious to eat. And more and more, the culture is changing towards healthy eating — they've even started selling raw cookies in Starbucks!

I've learned a lot about making healthy choices from Jeanine while we traveled together — she is a creative wonder when it comes to food. She also loves little indulgences every day, like a great piece of dark chocolate ("the weirder the flavor, the better"). She nibbles on things. (I love watching her eat. It's so fun — she's like a little kid.) She believes every day and every meal should be filled with celebration. In fact, in her mind, the day should BEGIN with celebration, and I have seen her do so with a decadent, delicately-made French pastry for breakfast. But she never overdoes it and she never goes unconscious or on automatic pilot. She'll taste, enjoy, one bite, two bites, and when she's done, she's done.

If she has to throw food away, she will. For example, Jeanine loves Doritos. One time on the road she bought a snack-size bag, ate about half, and the rest went in the trash. The bag says it's one serving, but Jeanine doesn't let a label tell her what a serving size is. She checks in with herself and knows how much to eat and when to stop. She eats only and exactly enough for enjoyment, pleasure and nourishment.

With restaurant food, the Yum Factor needs to be high, or Jeanine won't eat it. She doesn't just eat something because it arrived to her on a plate. Before ordering, she questions servers to find out how things are prepared. Once the food arrives, if something on the plate doesn't appeal to her, or doesn't taste totally fresh, she'll just skip it. She's not trying to be difficult, just honoring herself enough to make choices that will allow her to enjoy her food and feel great.

I have found that in restaurants, even the healthiest ones, you really don't know what goes into things — which is why I prefer to make meals at home. But I still love to eat out sometimes at great restaurants, so I follow Jeanine's example: I ask questions, and if needed I give detailed instructions about how I'd like something prepared. This way I can always find yummy and healthy things to eat.

I order dishes exactly the way I want them. If I need to, I'll pay extra for whatever changes I want to make. If something comes out and it's not how I ordered it, I'll ask them to make it again. Just recently I was at a "live juice" place where I ordered a green juice (with an added banana). I happened to be watching the guy make it, and suddenly I saw him squeezing something onto a tablespoon. I asked, "What is that?" and he replied, "Agave syrup," while he was putting it into my smoothie. I looked up at the menu board and said: "That's not on there." He said, "No, but we always put it in." And I said, "But it's not on the list of the ingredients. Can you please make me another one with no agave?" So, he put that one aside and made me a new one.

Before I worked with Jeanine, I never asked for what I wanted because I didn't know any better. I felt proud to be a person who could "eat anything" and not one of those picky people with so many food demands. I was annoyed by people in restaurants who asked for dishes to be made in a different way than what was listed on the menu. I used to be a waitress, so I also know that people who make menu modifications are a source of amusement and ridicule in the kitchen and among the wait staff. I never wanted to be THAT person who was the source of jokes in the kitchen. But then I realized: Why do I care what the wait staff thinks of me? This is my body and my life. Why am I ordering food that I don't really want, just so I can be an easy customer?

I have found a way to order food exactly how I like it — politely, with good humor and trying my best not to be difficult — so I will get what I really want with no sneaky ingredients added in. I have also learned that quite often even the cooks don't know what's in their ingredients because they come from a factory — so when I eat out, I try to find places that serve fresh and local. I prefer to eat everything simply, with no or little sauce. This is another choice I make to honor myself, to savor my food and keep my body feeling fit and vibrant.

Before this, I wouldn't go out of my way to find fresh, yummy, good food. I didn't know any better: I thought food was food. I thought food was calories, and that all calories were the same. I usually wanted to eat quickly because I had "so much to do" and needed to get eating out of the way, to get back to my to-do list. So, a bagel with cream cheese or a slice of pizza was my go-to meal. I would never have thought of driving an hour for a cup of great soup. That would have been a waste of time. Now, I see it as a mini-holiday in the middle of the day: the drive there, the scenery, the lunch, the drive back.

Now I make choices that respect my body. I choose whole, fresh, simple, organic, local. I eat plant-based, which to me means that the main ingredient is plants — fruits, vegetables, nuts and whole grains like quinoa — and then with this plant base, I'll add salmon, white fish, chicken, eggs. I stick to high-nutrient foods, straight from nature, bursting with sunlight. I no longer buy anything in a can. In fact, I choose to stay out of the middle aisles in the grocery store completely. I try to shop at small natural food stores or supermarkets that are connected to local farms, but sometimes I'll drive 90 minutes to Whole Foods. (I don't shop in the big super chains anymore — Hannaford's, Walmart, Shaw's — but even those places do have great choices in the outer edges of the supermarket.) I love farmer's markets when they are available. I live in New England, so when summer is over it's more difficult to find seasonal vegetables, but I still find them. I know all the best places and I travel there like it's a field trip.

When I'm at a party where other people serve me a big loaded plate or expect me to eat lots of unwholesome food, I will taste anything if I feel like it. I'll always try to bring a dish of something I love for sharing, so I can have some myself. When my mom's mac and cheese comes out, you bet I eat it! But only a few bites. I still love it, but I don't need a big bowl of it anymore. And I might still have some cake or cookies or pasta — but it's always a conscious decision to do so. I won't even try it if I can see that it's store-bought. I won't even take a bite. But if I see something that looks delicious and homemade, I'm curious. I'll taste it and check in with myself, "Is this the best cake on the planet? Do I love it?" If it is, I'll have more. Then I am present for the second bite — feeling for taste, texture, smell, enjoyment. Quite often, it's not the best thing I've ever had so a bite or two is enough and I'm done.

This summer, I'm spending 10 days walking the Camino de Santiago from Portugal to Spain, and I won't be bringing any food with me. But I'm not worried about it: I will just stay present and see what food choices there are. I make deliberate choices about what I eat, but I don't want to let it stop me from trying new things and going on adventures. I've been to Europe before and I found many restaurants and cafes serving food from the garden, so I'm sure I'll have no problem finding plenty of choices.

A WORD FROM JEANINE

Every day and with every meal, it's a good idea to remind yourself: You always have a choice. It may seem impossible to eat healthfully from a restaurant menu, for example. But, you can always ask your server for modifications or adjusted portions, even at a steak restaurant. Do you feel shy about asking for what you want when ordering food, maybe because you're afraid of what others around the table will think? Why? If your grocery doesn't stock a good selection of fresh fruits and vegetables, would you go out of your way to a different market with better choices? Why not? When you're at a party where you are served food that you would prefer not to eat, do you eat it anyway? Why? Start asking yourself these questions, and reminding yourself that you can always make choices that respect your body. In situations where you feel that you don't have a choice, brainstorm your options and write them down. Ask supportive friends and relatives for ideas and write these down, too. Then determine what options would work best for you.

FIT

EVICTING THE E-WORD

In addition to ditching the D-word, it's time to eject the E-word: Exercise. Or at least the kind of exercise programs and plans that promise results that never happen, because they are too exhausting, too boring or too troublesome for you to actually do them. These two words, "diet" and "exercise," belong in the self-torture chamber category — setting up expectations of a better tomorrow, while leaving you unchanged (but racked with guilt) today.

Packaged exercise programs are identical to diets in that they are meant to have a beginning and an end — a before and an after. And, as I'm sure you've experienced, they revolve around rules, and the guilt that you feel when you break them. So, I'm not exaggerating when I say I viewed "exercise" as torture. I was totally reluctant to start moving — I told myself I was too old, I was too busy, I was too tired, it was too much trouble.

On and off, I had tried the route of joining gyms, getting a personal trainer, making commitments, buying equipment, having a work-out schedule. But I could never stick to any of it. I made all sorts of excuses. If the trainer went on vacation or the gym was closed, my whole plan to exercise went out the window.

Even after I began losing weight and feeling heathier by changing my way of eating, I hardly changed my activity levels. People used to ask me all the time "Do you feel different? Do you feel amazing?" And the truth was that I didn't feel that different at all. I felt mostly the same — I was just a smaller size, wearing smaller clothes. Was I missing something? I felt like I was, but I still couldn't budge. I would read exercise and fitness books and look at all the photos of people posing on a yoga mat or doing something else athletic, and I would think, "YES. I want THAT life" ... and then nothing would happen. I might buy a yoga mat or a jump rope, use it once and then never again.

I saw myself as a couch potato, and I was one. (One day I even noticed a big indentation in the couch in the spot where I spent hours sitting every day, with the computer on my lap.) I lived mostly in my mind, and lost interest in the physical world and physical activity for years. In my teaching work, I have observed more and more people living this way — disconnected from their bodies, from nature, from physical activity — but it took me a while to recognize it in myself.

Deep down inside, I could recognize that I lacked balance. It's so weird that we sometimes know exactly what will make us feel great (and how simple it would be to accomplish), but yet we don't do it — we won't do it. Jeanine had encouraged me for years to jump rope or simply move at high intensity for just three minutes a day, but I wouldn't do it. It felt like way too much exertion. One jumping jack felt like too much. I know this sounds pathetic and lame, but there you go. I was so deep in resistance and stubbornness, with such an ingrained aversion to "exercise," that I had stopped moving, except to walk to the car, or go from room to room, from couch to chair to bed.

My husband, Bill Free, became my inspiration for living an active life. He had both his knees replaced, one in 2015 and the other in 2017, and I saw how dramatically different those two operations were for him. The first knee left him in pain for over one year. It took a long time to heal. (He didn't talk about his pain at that time — he only told me about it later.) We hadn't changed our eating patterns yet, and the only activity he managed was once a week when he went to his physical therapist and rode a stationary bike for 20 minutes. Before then, he had always been a very active person, but after that first knee surgery, he picked up my way of living — mostly staying inside, with minimal movement.

The second knee was a total different story. Bill didn't want to suffer like the last time, and was determined to heal quickly. He got off the pain pills in less than a month and bought a Spin bike for the house. As soon as the doctor gave him the go-ahead, he committed to riding the bike daily for 20 minutes. I watched him sweat every day. I saw his joy level increase. I saw his energy increase. Then I started to notice that he was being more active in general throughout the day, going outside more, finishing projects more easily, waking up earlier and going to bed later. Everything in his life seemed suddenly effortless. Coincidence? I don't think so. I witnessed Bill undergo a dramatic transformation — all from 20 minutes of exercise each morning.

I was inspired. Every day I would see Bill's energy and enthusiasm and say to him, "You are so awesome," and every day he would tell me how great he felt. Occasionally, without pushing, he would say to me: "Lisa, you would love this. It's so easy. Twenty minutes."

But still I struggled. I felt weak and powerless, and I felt guilty. I had Bill and Jeanine giving me motivation and inspiration to live in a new way, but in the end I knew that the kick-start had to come from within, from me. I had to take the time to look within and discover why I felt so reluctant to move and be active, and how to get past it. No one could do it for me. So often, I see health and fitness books that focus on the "after" picture of someone's transformation, and gloss over the "before." But I'm giving you an honest picture of my experience because understanding my negative, self-defeating attitude, my resistance toward "exercise" and getting physical, was the key for me to get past these issues.

So, I kept working at it, until finally I had my "aha" moment: In a flash of absolute clarity, I realized that I am a powerful being who was playing small, playing the victim, being weak and powerless. I'm not sure why I lived my life that way for so long, but I don't need to know. It doesn't matter. The point is that I had finally recognized that I HAD THE POWER to make new choices and live a new way, to break out of my routines and habits. I saw that I was letting weakness run the show and drive the car.

I realized that I needed to change what was occurring in my mind first, and then my body would follow. It's just like what I experienced with food: I changed my way of thinking about eating, and my actions followed. Often, we think that if we change our behaviors and actions (eat differently, lose weight, work out), then we will feel better, happier, sexier, stronger. But in truth it's the other way around: If you change how you think and how you feel FIRST, then your actions and behaviors will follow from that.

I decided that I was done with playing small. I knew that I had to get crystal clear on what I wanted my life to look like and, more importantly, what I wanted my life to FEEL like. And I knew it was an inside job. I reminded myself that I am here on this earth as a powerful being, to create, to serve, to love and to give, and that I no longer wanted to sit on the sidelines of my own life, beating myself up for not exercising. That's how the change in me began, honestly. I gave myself a break. I let go. I relaxed into it. I gave myself lots of space and permission to just BE.

Along with my new attitude, I knew I needed to come up with my own new motivation, something more inspiring than "lose weight" or "get in shape" or the dreaded E-word, "exercise." It was time for a new E-word that would honor the powerful, vibrant person I was: Energy. Instead of focusing on my body, I made my new goal to increase my energy — and flexibility, strength, stamina, endurance and balance.

I began to read inspiring stories and watch movies about dancers and athletes, and to get into their mindset and way of thinking. I would read interviews with Broadway dancers about what their lives were like. I got a subscription to Runner's World magazine, and would read about runners and their habits and routines. I got into their heads and into their lives. Then, I started thinking of myself as a professional dancer/athlete: No matter what, I had to "show up on the field," so to speak.

When you're on sports team or a dance squad, it doesn't matter if "you don't feel like it." The coach and the team are depending on you, so you're always there on time, early in fact, and ready to go. So, I decided to no longer give myself the option of not working out. No excuses, I had to do it. No more old routines, telling myself I was too tired, too busy. I had to be there on the dance floor, on the field. No more watching movies of other people being active while I sat on the sidelines.

The first step I took towards my new goal of living an active, vibrant life wasn't exactly the stuff that movies are made about: I moved off the couch and to a desk when working on the computer. This might seem like a nothing move towards fitness, but for me, it was everything. I made the decision — and followed it by action — and it was my first bold step towards a new life.

I didn't like it at first — sitting in a chair at a desk with my computer was not cozy the way the couch was. Everything in me screamed to move back to the couch, where it was comfortable. I noticed my resistance, watched my mind fighting with itself. I watched the thoughts come in, "This isn't going to work, you can start (sitting at a desk) tomorrow" — the same phrases my mind returned to again and again as I was making changes in my eating!

This right here was a huge revelation for me. To notice how hard my mind fought to stay in the old life and not change. But I was determined to change, and this was my first step: no more sitting on the couch for computer work. And sure enough, I felt my energy shift almost immediately. I noticed it took a different kind of energy to sit up straight in a chair vs. leaning back and slouching on the couch. This simple move was my firm beginning towards a new life!

My desk was piled high with papers and books, having become a storage space due to its non-use as a writing/work space. So, I cleared off the paper. I moved the books onto bookshelves. I got things organized. There was no turning back. The couch was still calling me, but I was determined to change my way of being from a couch potato to an energetic person who is vibrantly filled with love, more balanced, at peace, happy.

Taking this first step sparked something in me that I couldn't really put my finger on, but which felt very important. I had a big talk with my husband

and told him I was ready to change. I told him I wanted to be active. I wanted to go outside. I wanted to sweat. I wanted to change my routine. I felt like voicing my decision out loud to another person made it more real.

Little by little, I expanded my efforts to get out of my head and into my body. I wasn't trying to get in shape. I was just moving my body and being active every day in some way that felt good, gradually building up my activity levels over time. I started with small actions. Stretching for five minutes. Deep breathing. Bouncing up and down. Jumping jacks. Leg kicks. After so many years of inactivity, it felt like a whole new delicious experience to breathe deeply and feel this new energy bringing me to life again. I didn't need to go to a gym, or even go outside if I didn't feel like it. I just needed to move, in any way I could, and to do it consistently. I got rid of the idea that I was supposed to be an Olympian, and I focused on finding activities that felt joyful for me.

For the first time in a long time, I felt my energy creeping back. Ironically, where I would once tell myself "I'm too tired" and "I'm too busy" as excuses not to get up and exercise, the fact that I started moving soon gave me more energy to make time for being active, and everything else in my life. In a nutshell: Living an active life fills me with energy, and I accomplish more in a shorter period, effortlessly.

I could see and feel the changes in my body and my spirit. It's not that I felt like I was becoming a different person — more like I was becoming more of myself, like the person I had been as a child with the level of energy and enthusiasm I felt in high school and college. I began to remember how much I love dancing, and I started to connect with that part of myself again. It was like that part of me was always there, just waiting for me to engage with it again. It felt so good to move and to listen to music again.

Now I make time for regular activity throughout the whole day. I make a habit of getting up from the computer at least once an hour to just move — to dance or jump up and down or go outside and do some jumping jacks. I don't need to change into sneakers or workout clothes. I just concentrate on enjoying how my body feels when I breathe deeply, bounce up and down, do leg kicks. I recently started tap dancing, right in my home, and I love the feeling of being focused and centered on each step. It takes my mind off work and it's totally fun. I also make sure to sometimes take longer breaks for fun activities like long walks near the ocean or dance classes.

I love my new, active life. Working up a sweat gives me a burst of energy that lasts for hours. When I jump rope in the morning, I feel motivated and powerful — and I look at the clock and it's only 8 AM! I think, "Wow, this is amazing!" Then I head to the shower feeling like Wonder Woman. So, in the short term, working out gives me energy and clarity, and a feeling of accomplishment.

And, as I am consistently more active on a daily basis, I notice other, more long-term benefits. My breathing and circulation have improved, as have my sleep and digestion. My body is stronger, leaner and more sculpted — changes that make me feel powerful. I have more overall energy, and this helps me get everything done more easily and effortlessly. I also feel improvements in my posture, my focus, my mood and my concentration.

My new, powerful, active life has also led me to many unexpected benefits. It's given me an appreciation for what I am capable of physically: to walk, run, jump, bend and stretch. It helps me stay present in the moment, reminds me to breathe and gives me a big boost of oxygen which makes me feel happy, focused and energized. It makes me feel more playful, more alive, younger. I've also gained confidence: When I sweat, I feel like I can achieve anything and handle any challenge in life.

Another benefit: an improved level of gratitude. Being active clears my mind. It gets me out of my head, out of my stress, and I begin to see how much I have to be grateful for in my life. All that extra oxygen and blood pumping seems to get things flowing and moving, including my emotions and my creativity. I've noticed that, when I am active and connected to the moment, I am mentally inspired: All my best creative ideas come when I am running, dancing, playing, moving (or when I'm in the shower afterwards).

Maybe the best outcome of all is that I've started feeling like I'm more than my body's age. Most of us just unthinkingly believe what we hear all around us (from friends, from TV advertisements) — that you can't help but undergo a decrease in vitality as the years go by. But when you become active and have an inspired attitude — before you know it, your energy and vitality will go through the roof! You will begin to feel ageless, eternal and full of boundless energy.

All of these amazing changes unfolded for me when I moved beyond my old attitudes and habits with "exercise," and started to just be present in my body, to move it, to listen to it, to love it. You can do it too: Focus on improving your energy levels, your vitality, and your outlook, then start making small changes that will bring you to a vibrant, active life. Being fit starts with feeling strong and powerful, and then developing your body to reflect that fact.

A WORD FROM JEANINE

Scientists who have studied longevity in the Blue Zones — areas where populations are known to live longer, healthier lives than most — have found that these people typically lead active lives. However, that doesn't necessarily mean going to a health club, booking a personal trainer or engaging in any sort of traditional exercise regimen. Rather, they are naturally active in their environments, whether that means working in the garden or walking a distance to do errands. If you've had a sedentary lifestyle and would like to get more active, start with small, manageable fitness goals in terms of the frequency, intensity and duration of your activity. It can be as simple as getting up from your desk or chair once an hour to stretch your legs, or starting each day by climbing a flight of stairs or walking around the block. The important thing to keep in mind is to just keep moving every day.

FIT

MAKING FITNESS FUN

C hanging my deeply ingrained unconscious thoughts and patterns about fitness was a lot more difficult for me than changing my attitude toward food. I had started losing weight and feeling healthier through my dietary changes alone, but I hadn't yet experienced the level of vitality, aliveness and radiant health that I knew would be available to me if I became active as well. This is what I really wanted for myself. But even as I approached from this new mindset, I struggled with figuring out how to start living in a new, more active way.

I had not been consistently active for about 30 years. I would have "moments" here and there over the years, with bursts of activity and short-term gym memberships, only to slide back into the familiar patterns of sitting around inside, in front of the computer or television. I had become lethargic and slow-moving, and I knew that I didn't want to live out the rest of my life that way, but a lifetime of experience was telling me that exercise wasn't for me.

For most of my life, I thought being active meant exercising once a day (or a couple of times a week) for 30 minutes to an hour, and getting it out of the way. Do it and get it over with. When I did manage to get to a gym for a workout — walking on a treadmill or riding the stationary bicycle or climbing on the Stairmaster — I would feel bored. I'd try listening to music or reading magazines, but I was completely uninspired. It just wasn't fun for me.

Also, I always made workouts into a huge ordeal. I thought I HAD to push myself long and hard, so I would break into a sweat. If I did manage to get myself to the gym, there would be buckets pouring off me. (I could be very extreme back then.) I thought I needed special clothes, a daily workout routine, and a huge chunk of time to drive to the gym, get dressed, work out, take a shower, get dressed again and then drive home. So, most of the time I did nothing because I didn't have the time and I didn't want to go to all the trouble.

The bottom line was, physical activity did not come easily or naturally to me. I was extremely resistant to the thought of moving, working out and sweating — just thinking about sweating made my mind start racing with every excuse in the book not to do it. I couldn't see any appeal. I dreaded it.

When I started trying to figure out ways to motivate myself and get past these mental blocks, I realized that most of my unconscious patterns could be traced back to my childhood. As a child and into my early teens, I was naturally active. I couldn't wait to go outside and run and jump and ride my bike and play. But then, as I began developing, I noticed that people would watch me as I was jogging and running and biking outside. I didn't like being the focus of anyone's attention — I felt uncomfortable and exposed — so I retreated indoors.

After that, my main physical activity was school gym class, where for the most part the teachers would force us to get sweaty for an hour doing various sports and "exercises" that did not come naturally to me. I did not find this to be fun, like riding my bike or playing outside. It was torture. So, from this very early age I started equating "exercise" with a kind of punishment, enforced by others.

As I grew older, the message to exercise was a constant one, and it still brought with it feelings of reluctance, dread and guilt. I liked the idea of being fit, and enjoyed watching movies with people who were agile and alive, outdoors, going on adventures. I'd hear stories from people who surfed, biked, skied, hiked, canoed and paddle-boarded, and I would think, "I want to be THAT kind of person." But still I couldn't get my own heart into it. Every time I moved in that direction, I'd immediately want to go home, make a snack, read a book, watch a movie, check Facebook.

Thinking about my history with exercise finally led me to a breakthrough moment. What was missing from the equation? What would be the motivating factor that could get me over my reluctance and negativity? In the end, the answer was simple: HAVING FUN. Physical activity didn't have to mean what I always thought it did: arduous, boring exercise that happened at the gym.

I finally understood what Jeanine had been reminding me, through her words and example, throughout all the years of our friendship — that living an active life is about wonder and joy and curiosity, being a kid again, doing things you love for the enjoyment and pleasure of it. There is great satisfaction in being present IN your body — focusing on moving in it, feeling it move in the world, breathing deeply. Kids naturally play outside. They don't need to be told to go to a gym, to run, jump or skip. I had been looking at physical activity as a chore, and one that I was no good at. But no more: I needed to make fitness fun again.

I stopped thinking in terms of words like "workout" and "exercise" and "gym," and started thinking in terms of enjoyment — getting creative and discovering different ways to move that would appeal to my childlike sense of fun and adventure. I remembered that when I was a kid, I had dreamed of becoming a Rockette. So, I started dancing a little every day, practicing leg kicks — and eventually signing up for my first dance class.

I also rekindled my love for the outdoors. I live in one of the most gorgeous spots on the planet — in Maine near the ocean, near the mountains of New Hampshire, near lots of forest trails. Yet, for years, I rarely went outside, except to get in my car to drive to the grocery store or bookstore. There wasn't a good reason why — I had stopped being self-conscious in public years ago — except that seeing myself as an "indoor person" had become a bad habit. Now, I regularly make time for walks on the beach, exploring new hiking paths, or even just a 10-minute walk around the block.

Every day I get up from my desk, and either just walk outside for a few minutes or put a song on my iTunes and dance to that. One song usually leads to another song, and then another and then another. And suddenly I just danced for 10 minutes, it was totally fun, I'm sweating — but not dripping wet — and I feel happy. Instead of elementary school gym class (torture), it's more like recess, when you get to go outside and play for 15 minutes. I started thinking that way — 15 minute breaks, several times a day, to play.

These are the activities that I love, the ones that helped me to find the fun in being fit, and started me on the path to vibrant health. But there's no one-size-fits-all: The things that you enjoy might be very different. Think about what specifically is holding you back from getting active, and what will motivate you to change. Ask yourself, "What sort of things am I afraid of? What activities bring me joy?" And don't hesitate to get creative with it:

- If you are like me and you love dancing, make a playlist of great songs and take regular dance breaks at home, or even at work. Look for an empty office or conference room, or head to the parking lot for a few minutes.
- If like me you love the outdoors, do some research on nearby hiking trails, and try one you've never been to before. Or go for a walk in a different neighborhood, just for a change of scenery.
- If you feel shy about your neighbors watching you work out, go to a park instead, or invite a friend to work out with you, to boost your confidence.
- If you have fond memories of riding your bike when you were a kid, then think about taking it up again. Start slowly, or sign up for a cycling group and throw yourself right in.
- If you feel lonely and isolated, try signing up for just one beginner class at a gym or a yoga studio — anything that sounds intriguing. It's a great chance to meet other beginners who share your goals, or maybe even an inspirational instructor who can act as a guide in your journey to fitness.
- If you feel yourself falling into a rut, get unstuck by trying a change of scenery. Work out in a different room, or go for a walk somewhere

you've never visited before. Embrace the adventure of trying something new and get your creativity flowing. It's fun!

Fun may be subjective, but it comes in a million different forms. Once you've figured out the activities that are fun for you, then you can really get started in breaking the couch potato cycle. Trust me, it works!

A WORD FROM JEANINE

Your body was designed to move, not to sit still. Most young children don't have to be forced to run, jump, bike, climb, or skateboard. They simply enjoy being active. Rather than thinking of fitness as something you do only in a gym, while remaining sedentary the rest of the time, reframe your view of fitness as something that's part of your daily life, something that's fun, something involving play, something you look forward to. Find an activity (or more than one) that you truly enjoy — is it dancing to your favorite music, going for a brisk walk or scenic hike, jumping rope, martial arts? And think about planning more active social engagements — playing and being active with friends and family can make fitness even more fun.

SETTING GOALS

What does having goals have to do with changing your attitude to food and fitness? Everything. Goals are essential. In my life before, I was distracted and unconscious, with no clear goals as to what I wanted to achieve, other than a general desire to "lose weight" or "be thin." Because of this aimless wandering, I overate. You need clarity about what you want to accomplish so you can know where you are going, and then you can begin moving in that direction.

I had always dreamed of being a New York City Rockette, ever since I saw them in the Macy's Thanksgiving Day Parade on the television in my grandparents' house in Saratoga Springs, New York, when I was about 12 years old. I never pursued that dream, however, because I thought "that's for other people, thin people, real dancers." It was just a fantasy for me, nothing that I would accomplish in my lifetime. So, I went to college for hotel/restaurant management and received a BA in Communications. I worked for 10 years in marketing for a publishing company in NYC — a desk job from 9 to 5. I liked that job and I liked the people I worked with, but I didn't leap out of bed every morning in excitement to get to my desk. I forgot all about being a dancer.

As an adult, my goal in life switched over from "become a Rockette" to "lose weight." When and how do we diminish our goals? How is it that I went from wanting to dance on a stage in New York City to wanting to go down in pants size?

Let's face it, "lose weight" is just not that inspiring of a goal, and I think that's one reason why I had such difficulty with it over the years. It doesn't have a feeling to it. It didn't make my heart race. It didn't make me jump out of the bed in the morning in enthusiasm, like "Yay! I get to count calories today and be on a diet!" There is nothing inspirational about that. What's more, most of us who have "lose weight" as our goal don't really have a clear, definite picture in our minds about what we need to do to accomplish this goal.

As I worked with Jeanine, I realized I needed goals that made me feel excited and enthusiastic: embracing a whole new way of living and eating, being healthy and active by finding activities that are energizing and fun, finding ways to make my body feel vibrant and alive. I started to imagine myself as a dancer again, with a dancer's body and a dancer's life. I may never dance on a New York City stage as a Rockette, but I can still act like a Rockette in my mind, with daily habits that reflect the dancer within me.

When I started thinking of myself as a dancer, I instantly felt excited in a way I'd never felt when I simply wanted to "lose weight." As a result, I started doing things differently. As a dancer, I improved my poise and posture. I no longer thought of myself as a fat person. I thought of myself as an athlete with great, healthy eating habits. I read a quote that said: "A Rockette is an athlete dripping in diamonds." How great is that? So, I started thinking of myself as an athlete, which is not a way I had ever thought of myself before. Just like with food, when it came to movement and living an active lifestyle, I changed my mind, my outlook. I started thinking of myself as a professional dancer — even though I was only in my bedroom, practicing leg kicks.

Every goal begins with a thought and seeing it in your mind's eye. For me it was "I'm a dancer. I dance. I'm in the best shape of my life." It was that simple. I saw myself being fit and having lots of energy, carrying myself through the day — and through my life — like a dancer. I started buying Capezio black leotards to wear under blazers and with jeans, like I used to wear back in high school. I started watching dance movies and listening to music again. I felt like a dancer.

Just because you may never be quarterback for the Patriots (or look like Tom Brady), that doesn't mean you can't have an athlete's body. You can still work out like you are a quarterback for the Patriots, with the dedication of a pro athlete! Or you can be a yogini with a yoga body, flexible and strong with a great lung capacity. You can be anything you choose to be.

I love reading stories about athletes who have injured themselves but still keep working out. They still show up in any way they can, just to move and breathe and accelerate their healing process. They keep things moving because they always have their goal in mind: to get back on their feet and get back on the field, to get back on the stage, to get back on the bike.

Even once I had my new vision in mind, setting and achieving goals that would help me get there challenged me, and Jeanine's advice and guidance were crucial. It started with this important piece of wisdom — something very basic that had until now eluded me: "Lisa, you are in charge of your time. You are in charge of your day. You are in charge of your life."

This is common sense, right? Of course I am in charge of my time, but somehow it didn't feel that way. I was chronically addicted to my to-do list, rushing from one meeting to another, with an email box that was never empty no matter how much I tried to catch up. I was disconnected, unbalanced and not centered, spending a lot of time thinking about what I should be doing, but not actually doing it. I didn't take time to look inside and realize, oh yes, I AM in charge of my time, my day and my life.

The #1 thought running through my mind back then was "I'm busy." I said it to everyone, and I thought it non-stop. I'm busy, busy, busy. My schedule was filled with tasks, but I had no vision to where I was going. I was working hard trying to keep up, trying to hold my life and business together, but with no clear idea of what I wanted to accomplish or achieve. Every day was a race … to where, I don't know. I never took time to ask myself: What's the point of all this non-stop busy activity? Even my mother said to me, "Lisa, I'm tired of hearing you say, 'I'm busy' all the time. Stop it."

Jeanine has more on her to-do list than I do, yet she is relaxed and happy. I know that at the end of every day around 5 or 6 PM, she shuts down her computer and stops working. She lives in New York City where there's not a lot of quiet space. She has deadlines, travel, meetings — same as me — but a completely different attitude and outlook. She accomplishes all she wants to get done, easily and with grace — because she knows how to manage her time.

What Jeanine helped me to see is that my food/fitness difficulties were directly related to my habit of overcommitting and having no clear focus. I am a classic Type A personality who has a dozen different projects going on at every given moment in my life. I am naturally curious and want to try everything, but I noticed that instead of accomplishing things, I simply felt overwhelmed and was not completing anything. I had a bunch of half-finished projects. When I felt stressed (which was almost always), I turned to food, and kept on eating.

So, Jeanine asked me to identify what was important to me. What specific goals did I want to achieve and accomplish? What needed to take top priority in my day? I wanted lots of energy. I wanted my life to feel fun. I wanted to feel like a kid again: active, alive and vibrant. I wanted to go outside on a daily basis and simply enjoy nature. I wanted to walk the Camino from Portugal to Spain with my husband, Bill. These were some of my beginning goals. Jeanine encouraged me to write my specific goals down on paper and to keep them in a place where I could see them on a regular basis, to be reminded of what I want. Once I was clearer and more specific about what I wanted to accomplish, I was amazed how quickly things got done. It's usually only when we are distracted that small tasks take all day. "We all live in our heads. That's a bad place to live. Don't think about what you want to achieve and accomplish. Do it. Get out of your head." – Jeanine Barone.

Jeanine suggested this great exercise: Break up your day into short, 45-minute to one-hour segments. Know exactly what you are going to accomplish in that time frame and do nothing else. No email. No Facebook. No texting. No social media. Know what you are going to do and do it.

She also gave me another one that works perfectly with my Type A personality and drive to achieve: "Have a feeling of accomplishment first thing in the day." Many of the goals we set for ourselves could take months or years to achieve. But Jeanine taught me the value of setting goals for myself that I could accomplish before lunchtime! How awesome is that? You can choose something as simple as dancing or jumping rope for three minutes while waiting for the coffee to brew. Just get up out of bed and do it, and experience how incredible it is to have a feeling of accomplishment first thing in the morning.

The key is to find small goals that you can achieve *today*: Eat mindfully during one meal. Sweat for five minutes (or 10 or 30 or an hour — whatever you choose). Get up and move once an hour. This is do-able. The best part about setting small, achievable goals is that you will feel results straight away. You don't have to wait 10 days or three weeks or three months, like with your typical diet/exercise program. When I jump rope for three minutes first thing in the day, I feel energized all morning. I feel focused, clear and powerful. So, I enjoy the benefits immediately — and the feeling of achievement and accomplishment that comes with them.

Another key piece of advice I got from Jeanine: "I do not suggest weight-loss goals. Instead have lifestyle goals like: I'm going to be more mindful at meals. I'm going to be active for 15 minutes each day before going to work. I'm going to limit sugar. I'm going to try new fruits and vegetables to find ones I enjoy." Previously, I had always had a vague goal — lose weight — swimming around in my mind, but I would never do anything about it, or had no idea how to achieve it.

So, I ditched my goal of losing 40 pounds in three months (or dropping a fast 10, ASAP). I mostly stopped weighing myself. Jeanine advised: "If you are going to use the scale at all, do it once a week. Use it to see a trend and not to obsess about the numbers — numbers on a scale go up and down. Many people only pay attention to the number and don't factor in how they feel. Pay attention instead to how your clothes are fitting, how energetic you are, how mindful you are." These became my new goals.

Most importantly, Jeanine reminded me that true change c
overnight. It happens gradually. The big goals happen over ti.
small ones we can achieve every day. Jeanine said: "Think abou
saw real change in your life. You believed in yourself. You were
You stuck with it even when it was uncomfortable." Every day I ʋ
to getting at least one task done that would take me further to my ୍ɑɩ, and
I didn't procrastinate, even if it was something that seemed disagreeable at
first. I got it done, and that gave me a sense of accomplishment.

These are the keys to lasting change: You need to commit to a goal, you need
to believe in yourself and you need to do things to work toward that goal
even when you don't want to do them. So often we only want to do things
when they are easy. We fall into lazy habits, procrastination and unfocused
wishing for change. It's easier to live life in the passenger seat, but that's no
fun! It's more powerful and exciting to live in the driver's seat — to know
what you want and to go for it!

So, ask yourself, what do you really want? What is important to you? Spend
some time thinking about it. What needs to change in your life? Is there
some childhood dream you forgot about because it was too far-reaching?
Bring that memory back into your awareness. Choose goals that help bring
back the joy, curiosity, wonder and fun into your life. Let yourself dream.
Let yourself fly. Let yourself imagine and feel again, the way you used to do
when you were a kid.

Once you decide on the outcome you want, start taking steps in that direction.
Remember to be specific about what you want to change. Find small things
— you don't need a big overhaul all at once. What's one thing you can do
today? Take some time and find an answer. Write it down. Start with that
one thing and do it. You'll feel great! Then make a commitment to yourself
and stick with it. This new way of living must become a habit and a priority.
It's not an option. It's non-negotiable.

Remember to take time, every day, to envision that you are already at your
goal. Write down in words how you feel now that you have reached your
destination. This was especially helpful for me because, at first, I needed some

..agination to picture what it would feel like to be fit, energetic and healthy. So, like I said, I began to focus in my mind's eye: "I'm a Rockette." Then I would ask myself: What do I feel like? What do I eat? How do I move? What does my day look like? I'm vibrant, active, confident, focused and enthusiastic. I feel alive and happy, doing what I love, dancing. I'm still a writer, minister and spiritual teacher and I love that too, but I'm thrilled to be a dancer.

I focused on a goal of healthy eating — by that I mean unprocessed foods that don't come in a package. I looked in my cupboards and refrigerator — through the eyes of a happy, fit, healthy dancer — and realized immediately: This is NOT the kitchen of a happy, active, fit, healthy dancer. I went through all of my packaged and processed foods and asked myself, "Why am I eating something from a can that's been sitting on a shelf for a year or more? Is this going to be the most amazing thing I have ever tasted? If the answer was NO, I got rid of it. I tossed everything that had empty calories, along with everything that was not totally and utterly yummy. Straight into the trash (or the donation bin).

Just by taking this one step — achieving the small goal of cleaning out my cupboards — my life and attitude changed instantly. I felt a shift unlike any previous feeling when I started any "diet." This time I felt excited, inspired and hopeful. I thought: Well, THIS is do-able. This I can do. This will have immediate effects. No waiting.

I then set a goal of finding creative ways to eat healthy meals that are totally delicious. I made it into a happy game. I didn't want to eat just salads. In fact, I mostly don't like salads — I only really appreciate that "crunch, crunch, crunch" in the middle of the summer (and then I eat them every day). Typically, I prefer things that are warm or hot. So, I learned how to make a homemade lentil burger from real lentils, and perfected my recipe for salmon with asparagus. I made homemade soup from sweet potatoes or butternut squash, with chicken stock and some quinoa thrown in. That to me is a perfect lunch. And every time I had lunch, I accomplished my goal.

The trick is to have fun with it. I made it a priority to learn inventive, healthy ways to eat dessert: ice cream made in the blender from frozen bananas with cacao powder, raw chocolate coffee cheesecake made with raw cashews, coconut oil, almond milk and pecan-medjool date crusts. I taught myself to make "brownies" with raw walnuts, medjool dates and cacao powder, and lemon coconut raw cookies that are out-of-this-world good. In the process, I found out that eating healthy can be fun and delicious, and I accomplished my goal with every new recipe.

(I'll still occasionally eat a piece of cake made in the traditional way with sugar and flour, but more and more, I don't even want it — it makes me feel tired and sluggish afterward. I'm clear on my goal. I prefer my own raw desserts, which taste better and keep me energized.)

What I have learned through my own personal journey is that every action begins with a thought. When you act, speak and move like the person you want to be, you become that person. So, think about who you want to be, and what you want to accomplish in your life. Develop a vision for yourself that feels exciting, something to make you wake up every morning feeling inspired. When you have your goal in mind, speak from that place. This is your new self-talk. You're an athlete, an adventurer, a dancer, a world traveler, a person full of life, with boundless energy.

Write down your goal. Tell people about it. And work on smaller, specific steps to get you there. Even with the smaller goals, think in terms of feeling vibrant, alive, satisfied, and achieving something worthwhile. Make them specific and do-able, with clear-cut steps to take you closer to your larger vision for yourself. If your big dream is backpacking through Europe, or doing a half marathon or even a 5K walk — start with something simple like spending five minutes every morning walking briskly through your neighborhood. You'll return home every day having achieved your goal and knowing that your larger vision is that many steps closer to reality.

A WORD FROM JEANINE

It's well-established that if you want to achieve a goal, such as eating healthfully or becoming more fit, this goal should be both realistic and specific. For example, rather than saying, "I want to eat well," say instead: "I'm going to start by including fruit in my breakfast five times a week." Instead of declaring, "I need to exercise more," try: "I'm going to buy a jump rope and start jumping for 30 seconds, five times a week." These are very doable and specific goals. To make your goals even more doable, take baby steps. If eating fruit or jumping rope five times a week is too much, start with two or three times a week. Then once you have established a new routine, increase your goals bit by bit. Find out what works for you and re-evaluate whether it's still working over time. If not, try something else.

CHANGING YOUR SELF-TALK

As I think back over all the changes that have occurred during my amazing journey with Jeanine, if I had to choose the #1 single most important transformation in my life it would be this: I quit with the negativity going on inside my head and decided to like myself. I started to notice the constant excuses, self-criticism and guilt in my thoughts and the dismissive way I spoke about myself and my life to other people. This is called negative self-talk, and one day in a moment of clarity, I realized that it wasn't serving me or my goals. In fact, negative self-talk was actively hurting me and holding me back.

I'm a minister and spiritual teacher who trains people to notice their thoughts, feelings and beliefs and to decide to change them, and yet... I couldn't recognize my own blind spots when it came to my inner thoughts. My work includes a lot of travel, along with running an organization that has many programs, projects and staff, workshops, retreats, emails, interviews and creating new content and videos, and the most consistent thoughts running through my head on a daily basis were: "I'm so busy." "I'm tired." "I don't have time."

The organization was successful and growing, and I thought it needed my constant love and care. There was so much transformation happening for the people in our programs, and I needed to be there to support them, inspire them, help them all. What I didn't realize was that I was neglecting to give any love and support towards my own life and health. Sure, I would take a moment, here and there. But even on my "days off," I was still connected to the computer, thinking about work. I would read and answer emails late into the evening. I would get up earlier so I could get more done and try to catch up. There was always something that needed my attention (so I thought), and I did the best I could to stay on top of everything.

Because of all this external activity, I wasn't noticing my constant negative self-talk. Besides the "I'm so busy" mantra, what ran through my head was mostly criticism towards myself for how I wasn't able to be there for everyone. I also criticized myself for not enjoying life, for not exercising, for not being active, for not eating right. I truly thought I didn't have time. In my drive to help everyone else, I lost my connection with myself. I had no idea how much I needed to stop what I was doing and simply relax, listen within, take a break, take a vacation, have some fun and just play.

Through my work with Jeanine, I began to look inward and I finally saw it all. Privately, I was totally judgmental and critical towards myself, while cheering everybody else on. I truly believed that "I am what I am" — someone too busy to focus on my health, a homebody that likes to stay inside, eat comfort food and read. I tended to focus on all the ways I was failing, instead of trying to make positive changes.

During our weekly 30-minute phone calls, Jeanine was my constant cheerleader, encouraging me to tell her the areas where I had made a positive change. I would say things like: "Well, this wasn't a good week, I only worked out once" and Jeanine would point out: "Okay, first Lisa, drop the idea of 'working out' — this isn't about 'working out' — this is about being active, incorporating more movement into your life. And secondly, the way you just said, 'It wasn't a good week,' it's as if the whole entire week was a failure because you weren't active. Tell me how your week was great."

We had long conversations about my self-talk because it was especially self-destructive, and she would bust me on every phrase. I can't tell you how many times she would say "Lisa!" in an exasperated tone when I thought I was just "stating a fact." Besides the good old, "I'm too busy," the phrases I used the most were:

"I can't."

"I don't feel like it."

"I'm not there yet."

"There's something in my brain that makes me do it."

And the worst of them all: "I'm trying." (Jeanine especially did not like this one. She said: "'Try' is not a behavior.")

When I finally started to recognize my own judgmental self-talk, I decided to stop it. Quite honestly, my own over-critical, judgmental inner voice floored me. Jeanine would gently remind me that if I didn't take time to care for myself, I wouldn't be able to help anyone at all. She encouraged me to listen to myself, and we worked together on strategies to help me change my thinking. I began to notice my thoughts as they happened — to recognize when I would completely disqualify the positive and focus only on the negative — and then instead choose a more empowering thought that actually supports me. My favorite new, positive replacement thought that Jeanine gave to me: "I'm an active, vibrant Lisa Girl."

I love that word, "vibrant." I had never used it for myself. I had never viewed myself as vibrant, radiant or active, and thinking about these words was a lot more exciting for me than thinking about changing my diet and trying to lose weight, or how much I had to do — ideas that only depressed me. So, I started to think of myself as gorgeous, radiant, vibrant and alive, and something began to shift for me.

Here is what I learned through this transformation: The way we think determines the way we show up in life. Our thoughts become our actions. Our negative self-talk becomes a self-fulfilling prophecy.

You know what happens when you start to like yourself? Life gets easier. It gets fun. You are a whole lot gentler on yourself. One thing I did was start buying new clothes that fit me. For years when I bought something new and nice, I always "talked myself into" buying it a few sizes too small because of all the weight I needed to — and was definitely going to — lose. I would buy smaller clothes to "motivate" me.

My negative self-talk told me that I needed to keep wearing the baggy, oversized, worn-out clothes that fit me for now and treat myself once, and only if, my ideal life arrived. Ironically, that same voice also told me I didn't need to work out and exercise or be active. It told me I was fine just the way I was: "You can't help who you are." And I would nod in agreement. Then I would just continue to sleepwalk through life, working, staying indoors, eating cheese nachos.

Take the time to look inward and become aware of your own negative self-talk. Begin to recognize when and how you put yourself down. Notice how easily you talk yourself out of certain things (getting active) and how effortlessly you talk yourself into others (a second or third helping of food when you're already full). Another good method is to listen to what you say about yourself to others: Pay close attention to how you refer to yourself, how you describe yourself — especially during conversations about your body, your physical fitness and the food you eat. Are your thoughts inspired by your own authentic voice? Do they give you guidance, protection, care and encouragement? If not, then replace them with ones that do.

I have discovered that I can choose thoughts that support me and the life I want to live. So now, I make sure my self-talk is positive and loving. I'm active. I get things done easily and quickly. I love my life. I take long, leisurely breaks in the middle of the day. I go outside and explore. I take holidays. I get off the electronics — "off the grid" — for days at a time. I'm an active, vibrant Lisa Girl.

A WORD FROM JEANINE

Are you aware of how you speak about yourself both in your own thoughts and out loud to other people? Think about whether these statements sound familiar: "I'll never lose weight; Losing weight is hard; I hate exercising; I'm not naturally athletic; I ate a few cookies, now my eating plan is ruined and I might as well give up; Healthy food tastes terrible; I don't like any vegetables." Negative self-talk like this can obstruct your path to a healthy lifestyle — in fact, it can stop you before you even get started. Pay attention to any negative thoughts, make note of them, and then refute them, talk back to them, reframe them or phase them out. Instead of thinking you're a failure because you slipped up, focus on the progress you've already made and that you will make in the days ahead. Instead of saying that you hate all vegetables, say that you're going to try new ones or new recipes to prepare them in unexpected, yummy ways. Instead of telling yourself that you're no athlete, focus on appreciating what your body can do and the increased energy levels you get from having a more active lifestyle.

——— AWARE ———

MAKING YOURSELF #1

It's been a long journey to get to where I am today. Many of my friends and students only see the external changes (60 pounds in 10 months) and have asked me to share my eating plan (as I've done earlier in this book, although it's not so much a plan as a way of thinking). But the full story is not quite so simple. It took me years of doing inner work — examining my beliefs and patterns of thinking, being willing to see things differently, and working to change my mind and find balance — before this inner work "suddenly" began to reflect in the physical (my food choices, my body, my appearance). The real changes I made were completely internal. Once I shifted my thinking, the transformation that happened seemed miraculous. I became deliberate in finding out the causes of my overeating and overcoming them, and external effects followed very quickly.

One of the most important steps I took toward healing my self-sabotaging attitudes around food and my body was the conscious decision to "Make Me #1." Jeanine came up with this idea for me after several phone counseling sessions in which she saw that I was putting myself second, third, fourth and, sometimes, last. Out loud, I agreed with her because I could grasp on an intellectual level that making self-care a priority was exactly what I needed. If you've ever taken a flight, you know that the first rule in an emergency is to put the oxygen mask on yourself first before you attempt to help anyone else. Otherwise, you might not be able to help anybody. This same rule holds true in life, and yet I was not following it.

Making Me #1 is about recognizing and honoring your own self-worth. It is about putting yourself first in your own life, about loving yourself and caring for yourself.

For a long time, I was very disconnected from my life, very disconnected from my body. In this world, many of us are taught that it's selfish to put ourselves first. We get the message that we need to be givers and helpers to others — which is all fine and good, but not at the expense of ignoring our own needs.

It was like that for me. From an early age, I felt an instinctive need to take care of other people. I was a happy child, full of joy and wonder, but I could see that people around me suffered. I believe a lot of children have this kind of instinctive, intuitive wisdom, as well as a natural ability to give effortless, unconditional love. I somehow understood that I had the ability to calm a situation with my presence, even at five years old. I was nicknamed "the peacemaker," and told I was a calming personality who people liked having around. I embraced that identity, and out of this evolved a whole belief system based around my responsibility toward others. Without conscious awareness of my feelings, my instinct told me it was up to me to take care of everyone and everything.

For most of my life, I would treat my own needs as unimportant. I felt that other people needed me more, and that I could help them achieve their goals. I could be there for them, to bring joy, love and sunshine. I see this pattern in many of my students as well. Because we put other people's needs in front of our own, the only ways we find to take care of and comfort ourselves are quick fixes like food and mindless distractions — going unconscious instead of taking the time to look inward and discover what we really need.

As an adult, I naturally gravitated toward work that would allow me to help others. I started an organization that was thriving, with a growing team, and I was supporting and counseling people every day. But the problem was, my health was failing. My energy level was practically at zero. I felt overwhelmed all the time. My eyes burned from constantly staring at a computer screen for too many hours each day. I was stressed out, tired, low energy, overweight and overeating.

I can't tell you how often I put some time for myself on the calendar (go to the gym, take time off), and then someone would call and NEED ME. So, of course, I would rearrange my schedule. I felt pride in the fact that I was never late for appointments with other people — in fact, I was usually early, and sometimes I would show up with a thoughtful gift. But did I treat myself with the same kind of care and respect? No! I would cancel my own appointments with myself at the last minute without thinking twice. I honored other people's schedules, but not my own. I didn't value myself enough to do so.

At the time, I thought I was taking fairly good care of myself. Every morning, I'd write for a little while (a journaling practice I'd been doing for years called Morning Pages, created by writer Julia Cameron). Every night, I'd try to fit in a bath or some quiet reading time before bed. Looking back now, I see that my self-care plan added up to maybe an hour total at the beginning and end of the day — and I wouldn't pay an ounce of attention to myself in between. I would go mostly unconscious throughout the entire day's activities: emails, work-related projects, reacting to all the many different requests that are sent to me on a daily basis. I ate breakfast and lunch while working in front of the computer. I rarely went outside. I had a dinner break with my husband Bill — usually a heavy meal of "comfort food," with huge portion sizes. Then I would often feel exhausted after these big meals, not energized or rejuvenated.

Deep down I knew that I was overloaded and overwhelmed, but I kept telling myself that sometime down the road, later, in the future, I would be able to relax, rejuvenate and take better care of myself and my body. When my life eventually slowed down, I would be able to make some healthy changes. But here's the thing: My life wasn't slowing down. It just kept getting more and more chaotic and fast-paced. I was traveling all the time, getting invitations to speak and teach, and new people were signing up for our online programs every day.

I never really paused long enough to see that my own life was zipping by me in a blur of stress and guilt. My work just kept getting busier and busier, until finally I crashed: My wake-up call came in the form of a severe illness while on a teaching trip in Guatemala in March 2016. It brought me to my knees, and I knew something had to change. I realized: This is my life now. It's not later. It's now. I had to start making ME my #1 priority, so that I could finally take care of my health, my life.

In the beginning, I struggled. When I first started saying "no" to people, I felt terribly selfish. The voice in my head screamed, "But they need you!" It was an uncomfortable feeling to put myself before my friends, marriage and work: I had tremendous guilt about letting people down. Some people even told me they were disappointed in me. One friend called me selfish and self-centered — not a good friend — and then she broke up with me. Previously, this would have had me running for the cookies, but instead I took a breath and remembered that this was my life and that my health was my priority. I reminded myself that I needed my own friendship. I needed to stick with my commitment to put myself in the #1 spot, and stop spending all my energy on pleasing everyone else.

Through it all, Jeanine's counseling was essential. She helped me realize that the way I was eating was not taking care of me — in fact it was doing the exact opposite. She taught me that real self-care involves giving yourself time to relax and recharge, listening to your mind and your body, making changes that support them and being gentle with yourself. I began starting every day with a mantra Jeanine gave to me: "I am always good to myself." The key word here is "always." I am ALWAYS good to me. In the past I would put myself first, maybe once a week or once a day. The "always" is a game changer. Now, I remind myself to be good to me, all the time.

When I began taking charge of my time, I discovered how awesome it feels to live life with intention, and not feel powerless over my schedule anymore. Now, I prioritize my days to include more leisurely mealtimes, so I can enjoy the experience rather than spend my time working through meals. I also make it a point to allot time for physical activity, play, rest, movies and fun.

Morning Pages, a longtime practice for me every day when I wake up, was probably the best thing I did for myself over the years. In her work, Julia Cameron also suggests a Weekly Artist Date — giving yourself a few hours every week to take yourself out "on a date" to explore and discover, to do something fun. In all my years, I had never once managed to honor the Weekly Artist Date, although I had tried to schedule it for myself occasionally. So, I started to put it on my calendar, and I made it a practice to never break this appointment with myself.

As I started taking better and better care of myself, I started feeling great. I was more present than ever before. I was calmer, happier, gentler and more relaxed. My creativity started coming back. I felt alive, with the vitality creeping back into my body. People noticed the change in me. They would say, "You're different," and I'd know that it was meant as a compliment.

Of course, I still pride myself on the work I do to care for others — it's incredibly important to me to feel like I am helping and doing good in the world. But now I don't do it at the expense of my own body, mind and health. I take the time — and I make the time — to take care of myself, to be in the moment and to pay attention to my own needs. Making yourself a priority is the key to it all, so put yourself in the #1 spot.

A WORD FROM JEANINE

Do you devote time and energy to helping and caring for others, but feel guilty when you do the same for yourself? Studies have found that people who take time to care for themselves are more likely to maintain a healthy lifestyle, including a healthy body weight. That means carving out time in your life to devote to your own well-being, whether that means taking dance classes, enjoying walks outside, regularly shopping for an array of fresh fruits and vegetables or even taking up a hobby you left behind because you were "too busy." Caring for yourself isn't selfish behavior, but rather self-care behavior: It's not that you are the only priority, but rather the top priority. Make a commitment or promise yourself to do something healthy, something that brings you joy or happiness, every day.

AWARE

LOCUS OF CONTROL

O ver the past couple of years, I have learned many lessons. I've learned that I am 100 percent responsible for my life: It's me who has to do the work; no one else is going to do it for me. I've learned that in the middle of chaos, I can always choose joy and peace over pain and confusion. I've learned that the most beautiful life is about balance, which includes lots of moments of play, adventure, curiosity and enjoyment. I've learned to care for my body. I've learned to make food choices that support my vision of a vibrant, active, healthy, fit life. I've learned to be gentle with myself because let's face it, life is about living, not about strict rules or being perfect. Life is meant to be messy, disorderly, disruptive — and that's what makes it so fun. It's about listening to what you really want on a moment-by-moment basis and honoring that inner voice.

Most of all, what I've learned is that I'm in charge of my attitude. I'm in charge of the way I feel. I'm in control of my thoughts, my words, my emotions. I'm in charge of what I put in my mouth and eat. I'm in charge of how active I am. This consciousness can be called an *internal locus of control:* the realization that *I* am the determining factor of my life. I choose how my day is going to be, I choose how my life is going to be: how I respond to events during every day will determine how I will live my life.

This idea of internal/external locus of control came from psychologist Julian Rotter in the 1950s. The underlying question is: Do I control my life or does something else (like God, fate or some other external force) control it?

My internal locus of control is what makes me self-motivated. I eat healthfully not because some book has told me to eat healthfully, but because I know how awesome I feel when I do. I'm a healthy, active person and I don't need a trainer or a program to be the most vibrant, alive person I can be. I don't need gimmicks, prizes, awards or rewards. I don't need stickers or congratulations from other people for a job well done each week that I eat right, and I don't need to reward myself. I'm self-motivated every day because that is the reward in itself. That's the prize.

People with an external locus of control tend to blame outside forces for how things are going in life. They allow people, places and things to determine how they feel and how they live. When it comes to weight loss and fitness, having an external locus of control means depending on things outside of yourself for motivation and help in making decisions. You need someone or something else to tell you what to do, what to eat, how to eat, when to eat. And when you depend on a diet program, you stop trusting in the wisdom of your own inner guidance. With an internal locus of control, you begin to trust in that still small inner voice.

With an external locus of control, you need rewards or punishments to stay on track. You need positive reinforcement/encouragement from other people to help you stay on a diet or a daily fitness plan. But think about it: What happens when you're not able to get to the gym or get to the meeting? What happens when the person who has been telling you, "You're awesome! Keep going!" suddenly isn't there for you in the moment when they roll out the dessert tray?

Another example of having an external locus of control is when you say, "I can't because...." I can't because it's too hot. I can't because it's too cold. Because the gym isn't open, or because it's too far away, or because I can't afford a membership. Because the kids are home. Because I'm too busy with work. How do you end this sentence? What's your excuse? What is your why? What's the thing you are blaming? Be aware of it. Outside forces will always be there. Always.

Jeanine told me that most people with a strong internal locus of control also have a high self-worth and a great ability for motivation and action. They do things for themselves because it feels good.

Before I realized my own value, in truth, my self-worth was at the extreme low end of the scale. I thought that losing weight would change this. But, as Jeanine pointed out to me, self-worth has nothing to do with changing your body: It's about changing your mind and attitude, which can be done any time you choose. And now would be a great time to make that change.

When you begin to value yourself, everything begins to transition. You show up in a new way. People with a high self-worth don't do things because they "have to" or they "should." They do it because they want to, because they love it, because they have found an internal motivation that drives them and that is a reward in itself.

Jeanine said to me: "Lisa, be a person who takes charge. You are in control of what you put in your mouth and how active you are." That was the best advice ever. It helped me realize, hell yeah, I'm in charge. I decide what happens with my life.

This was not always true. For years, I felt I had no control. If mac and cheese was around, IT was in control. If cake was around, I was its slave. When I went on a diet, I would bribe myself with gifts to stay on track, or reward myself with a hot fudge sundae if I lost X number of pounds, which is just about the dumbest idea ever when I think about it now. But for most of my life, this was logical thinking to me. I would promise myself a $100 shopping spree for every 10 pounds lost. I would join online weight loss communities so that I would have other people's encouragement to keep going.

I used to tell myself that I could only work out when the gym was open, or when the weather was good (not too hot and not too cold), or when

I had money to hire a trainer or buy a piece of equipment. I couldn't exercise when I traveled because I was too busy, and because of the horrible conditions in hotel gyms. Sometimes I didn't have my sneakers or socks with me. Sometimes there was no gym, so what was I supposed to do then? Sometimes it was raining outside, or snowing. Sometimes I had scheduled breakfasts, lunches and dinners, and not a single moment of free time. Talk about an external locus of control!

So be aware if you are blaming your diet, the weather, other people, your living situation, your problems, your metabolism or your genes for your lack of results. You don't have to eat something just because someone spent hours cooking it, or because their kid spent hours baking it. You don't have to eat three plates of food at the buffet just so you can get your money's worth. You can take back your power.

In my work with Jeanine, I started looking at all the things that side-tracked me. I made an effort to notice the list of things I thought I'd need to lose weight, get healthy, be fit and be active. Jeanine kept telling me: "You don't need all that stuff, Lisa." And she was right. I didn't need another diet. I didn't need exercise equipment. I didn't need a gym membership. I didn't need a trainer. I didn't need fancy kitchen appliances. I didn't need to go to a spa. I didn't need to measure my food or count calories or fat grams. I didn't need to wait until summer or until Monday to get started. I had everything I needed, now.

The way I began to process my power over my food and fitness choices was by relating it to how I stopped drinking alcohol. I quit drinking and smoking in 2001 because it had become a problem for me. I haven't touched a drop of alcohol or picked up a cigarette since, and I won't touch alcohol even if it's the only thing to drink. The bottle can be right there in front of me, someone can pour me a glass of wine, and I won't touch it. It's not a temptation for me, I simply don't want it. While traveling through France with Jeanine, every night our hosts would serve wine and on one occasion I was told I HAD to drink it, that it was rude not to. I didn't touch it. Why? Because I didn't let things outside of me control me.

Nobody can guilt me into drinking alcohol, and no one can guilt me into eating unhealthy.

Now, when someone puts a basket of bread on the table at a restaurant, it's totally fine to me. I don't need the server to take it away. Just because bread is on the table doesn't make me go powerless: Bread is not the boss of me. I don't have to eat it just because someone brought it to me, or to make my dinner companion feel more comfortable eating it. I may or may not have some, depending on how I feel in that moment. Normally I'll just skip it because it's processed, packaged bread that was made in a factory — it's just a whole lot of empty nothingness to me. But sometimes — if it's homemade (or the baker is from Italy or France, or trained in Italy or France), I'll go for it. If I do eat the bread, I have one bite and check in with myself. "Is this good? How's the Yum Factor? Do I love it? Do I need another bite? Do I want another bite?" I'm totally aware of what's going on. I don't go unconscious. Internal locus of control, all the way.

If you ever think, "I can't jump rope (or skip or hop or bend and stretch) because I don't have anywhere to do it," think again. Having an internal locus of control means knowing that you can always find a few minutes to move, no matter where you are. You can dance or jump or run in place for several minutes in your bedroom, in a hotel room, even in the hallway or out on the street. And so what if people see you — when you worry about what other people think about you, that's an external locus of control again.

Have you ever seen those boxing movies or high-school football movies where the hero is a down-and-out nobody slacker/loser and he decides he is going to change his life? What happens next? He's up at the crack of dawn and outside running. In the rain. In the snow. He's jumping rope wherever he is. He doesn't care who's watching. He's doing it. He's going all the way. Nothing can stop him from being the best. And we're all sitting there on the couch, totally inspired by this guy. But he's got nothing special over any of us — except a vision for greatness and the drive to go for it. All you need is to have a vision of greatness, and to get past the excuses and live it.

I've learned that nothing has power over me to derail my fitness goals or food choices. I'm the boss of me. I'm in control. I'm in the driver's seat. I know where I'm going. I know what I want. I know how to accomplish it. And nothing is getting in my way … nothing. That's how I lost 60 pounds with what felt like no effort. Every day I exerted my own power to make food and fitness choices and I was consistent at it.

I wasn't perfect at it. But I was consistent in going forward with my new way of living. I still eat mac and cheese (and totally love it), but now I decide that I can have a small portion and be completely satisfied. I don't let one bad food choice derail me for the entire weekend (or month) like I used to, I get right back on track. In fact, I stopped naming certain foods "bad choices" because that's having an external locus of control again. Sometimes I just want bread with butter and strawberry jelly or a piece of cake or pasta with cheese and so I have it. No guilt. No judgment. Total enjoyment. But I also know, okay, I am not eating this way every day.

That's an internal locus of control. The food is not in control. The weather is not in control. The location is not in control. The diet program is not in control. YOU are in control.

Remember, you are unstoppable. You are in charge. Nothing whatsoever has the power to stop you from being happy, alive and radiant.

A WORD FROM JEANINE

The term "locus of control" refers to your perception as to who is in charge of your life. People with an internal locus of control believe they have control over their lives; those with an external locus tend to attribute the circumstances of their lives to outside factors. Most of us fall somewhere in the middle: Think of it as a continuum between high-internal to high-external and everything in between. Studies have found that people with a high locus of control are more likely to engage in physical activity and to successfully lose weight than those who feel that, for example, that their genes are to blame, that they just have naturally low energy levels, that their busy lives or family demands won't allow them to live a healthy lifestyle, or maybe it's just their fate to be overweight. Do any of these excuses sound familiar? If you feel powerless over your life, try to look at all the choices — even tiny ones — that are available to you as you go through your day. Though they may seem trivial, making regular, small, healthy choices will get you in the habit and allow you to feel more confident in taking charge of your life. Rather than focusing on what you can't control, be attentive to what you can: your thoughts and your responses to situations. If this is a struggle for you, try to connect with the proactive people in your life, observe how they approach things and learn from their example.

EPILOGUE

When I started working with Jeanine in September 2014 to change my attitude toward food and fitness, I could never have imagined that four years later in June 2018 I would walk 150 miles along the Portuguese route of the Camino de Santiago — and do so with a sense of ease and joy. (In 2014, I was NOT that girl. Rather, I was a sit-by-the-beach and a relax-in-the-sand kind of girl, reading inspirational self-help books, hoping that my excess weight would magically dissolve.) And, yet, that's exactly what I did with my husband, Bill, and 20 friends. We walked 150 miles in 14 days.

This trek showed me how radically my attitude toward myself and my life has transformed since my walking trip in Brittany, France with Jeanine in June 2015 (where every day felt like a physical struggle to put one foot in front of the other). It was this France trip that opened my eyes to my poor level of fitness. It showed me that something had to change — I couldn't just keep hoping and praying for a miracle. I had to BE the miracle and do the work. On the Camino, I put into practice what I had learned: That I'm the agent of change, and that any limitations or obstacles I perceive are created by me. I felt first-hand how powerful, strong and healthy I am; the abundant energy I have to race up mountains like a little kid, to hike through forests, to walk along the ocean; and I was able to enjoy it all without being distracted by the weight of my body and the heaviness of my old thoughts. Often people measure "success" and "results" by counting numbers on the scale or inches or clothing size. I got to measure my results by enjoyment of life. My biggest "ah-ha moment" on the Camino was realizing what Jeanine has been telling me all along: that it's the journey that's oh-so important, rather than the destination.

For most of my life, I wanted to get to the destination as fast as possible with the belief that something wonderful would happen after that. For years, I thought that life would begin once I lost 40 pounds and got in shape. What I now know is that *every* moment is "that something wonderful," and that I simply have to be present in the moment to enjoy it. On the Camino, I decided that I wanted to stay outside (in nature) all day, enjoying picnics in the sunshine along rivers, leisurely cups of coffee in cafes with friends, putting my bare feet in the grass, and sharing an apple with almond butter with whoever was with me. Why rush to the hotel? This is my life: enjoying and paying attention to my experiences, appreciating the beauty around me.

I am now aware of my thoughts and how they affect my experiences. At one point during the Santiago trek when it was pouring rain, I was all set to catch a cab and rush back to my warm, dry hotel room. This was the old Lisa. But I stopped for a moment and checked within. I knew that walking in the rain was part of the adventure. So, I made a decision to continue on the trail no matter what, and it turned out to be one of my favorite parts of the trip. We all got soaked. We laughed the whole way. We took photos. We took our time, enjoying the coolness of the rain and the sun filtering through the clouds.

On this trip, I became aware of little things that had escaped my notice my entire life: the aroma of pine trees, the sound of my sandals crunching dry branches and leaves, the slipperiness of wet rocks in the mountains as I climbed, the warmth of the sun radiating through the dense forest, the way different muscles worked in my back, legs and ankles based on the terrain. How did I not notice any of this before? Because I was stuck in my mind with thoughts of self-hatred; I was too busy putting myself down. Now that I am no longer engaged in self-sabotaging thoughts, I am able to see what was always right in front of me. I also find myself feeling deep appreciation for things I used to take for granted: my ability to breathe, my capacity for gratitude and the power to be delighted by every little thing. This is my life now, a world full of wonder and discoveries in my environment and inside me.

I love knowing that I'm the one who decides what to eat. Being in another country, out of the familiar territory of my kitchen, I became aware of how far I had come not only with my fitness but also with food. The food options were completely different from what I was used to at home, but I was mindful of making choices that would nourish my body and, equally important, that had a high Yum Factor. I'm no longer a victim to my thoughts that told me to eat triple portions. Those thoughts don't control my behavior. I'm in charge.

Unlike all of the previous diets and fitness plans I've tried — only to revert back to my old habits — I know there is no going back to the way I used to be. The changes in me occurred gradually over time and there was nothing extreme in what I did. I simply took the time to examine and evaluate my attitudes and beliefs, and made small, consistent changes toward healthier food choices and a conscious decision to be active. That's it. Years ago, I would never have taken this route as I was focused on fast results and a change on the scale. When I see my life now, I'm happy I took this slow path: It's what led me to be vibrant, healthy, active, joyful and full of gratitude.

AFTERWORD

Throughout this book, I've mentioned the importance of "The Yum Factor" when it comes to the food that you choose to eat. But the Yum Factor is about more than food: Your meals should be yummy, but so should your physical activities, and so should your life! Remember, there is no one-size-fits-all: What's Yum for me might not be that way for you. So, listen to your body, determine what it needs and then love it in the best way possible. Finding your own personal Yum Factor is the first step toward living a vibrant life filled with joy.

47402624R00063

Made in the USA
San Bernardino, CA
12 August 2019